AGING AND CLINICAL PRACTICE: MUSCULOSKELETAL DISORDERS

A Regional Approach

AGING AND CLINICAL PRACTICE

Series Editor: Isadore Rossman, M.D.

INFECTIOUS DISEASES: DIAGNOSIS AND TREATMENT
Thomas T. Yoshikawa, M.D.
Dean C. Norman, M.D.

MUSCULOSKELETAL DISORDERS: A REGIONAL APPROACH
Robert R. Karpman, M.D.
John Baum, M.D.

AGING AND CLINICAL PRACTICE: MUSCULOSKELETAL DISORDERS

A Regional Approach

Edited by
Robert R. Karpman, M.D.
Chief of Orthopedics
  Maricopa Medical Center
Director of Phoenix Orthopedic Residency Program
  Phoenix, Arizona
Clinical Associate Professor in Surgery
  University of Arizona
  Tucson, Arizona

John Baum, M.D.
Professor of Medicine and Pediatrics
  and of Preventive Family and
  Rehabilitative Medicine
School of Medicine and Dentistry
University of Rochester
Rochester, New York

IGAKU-SHOIN   New York • Tokyo

Cover Design by M'NO Production Services, Inc.
Typesetting by Arcata Graphics/Kingsport
Printing and Binding by Arcata Graphics/Halliday

Published and distributed by

IGAKU-SHOIN Medical Publishers, Inc.
1140 Avenue of the Americas, New York, N.Y. 10036

IGAKU-SHOIN Ltd.,
5-24-3 Hongo, Bunkyo-ku, Tokyo

Library of Congress Cataloging-in-Publication Data

Musculoskeletal disorders.

   (Aging and clinical practice)
   Includes bibliographies and index.
   1. Musculoskeletal system—Diseases.   I. Karpman,
Robert R.   II. Baum, John.   III. Series.   [DNLM: 1. Bone
Diseases—in old age.   2. Joint Diseases—in old age.
3. Muscular Diseases—in old age.   WE 140 M9851]
RC925.M854   1988   616.7   87-16847

ISBN: 0-89640-138-3 (New York)
ISBN: 4-260-14138-4 (Tokyo)

Printed and bound in U.S.A.

10 9 8 7 6 5 4 3 2 1

Preface

Musculoskeletal Problems in the Elderly—A Regional Approach to Diagnosis and Therapy

The most frequent rheumatic disease is osteoarthritis; it is largely an illness of the elderly. National statistics for office visits of patients 75 years old and over list "osteoarthrosis and allied disorders" as the fourth most frequent diagnosis, following hypertension, chronic ischemic heart disease and diabetes (1).

It can be seen from this information that as the population continues to age, we will be increasingly faced with the diagnosis and treatment of a large geriatric population with musculoskeletal disease. As our skill with surgery improves and new and better prostheses are developed, we will be able to better maintain our elderly population in a functional state. Our intent here is to help primary-care practitioners maintain their patients in optimum musculoskeletal status. This book will also be of use to house staff and medical students, with their needs for improving diagnosis and therapy in the geriatric population. Our intent is to combine in a succinct manner rheumatologic, orthopedic and neurologic concepts in discussing musculoskeletal disorders by a regional approach rather than as separate entities. We believe that this approach will be the most useful one for practitioners who see patients in a primary-care setting.

Musculoskeletal complaints are more difficult to identify in the elderly than in the young. For instance, in young patients, back pain is more often associated with occupational insults and is more frequently seen in men. With advancing age, there is a shift of complaints of back pain toward women. Also accompanying these area-specific problems is a higher likelihood of other body systems and musculoskeletal structures entering into the complaint pattern.

Primary-care physicians may be faced with the dilemma of having problems with not only the diagnosis but also often with deciding which specialist to use for referral. Particularly with back pain, a number of questions arise. Does the patient have osteoporosis alone, or has a vertebra collapsed? Could the problem be Paget's disease localized to the spine? What about diskitis? Osteoarthritis is a major problem but because a radiograph in this age group would show this change as a matter of course, another true cause of the patient's complaints could be missed. Referred pain or pain in the limbs raises the possibility of local pressure at an outlet or spinal stenosis or an intraluminal tumor.

Who will provide the most help in diagnosis and therapy? In this book, we have depended mostly on the expertise of orthopedists and rheumatologists.

Indeed, the discussion herein is directed as much to them as to primary-care physicians who want to learn more about the problems that they will be facing to an increasing degree. Because of cutbacks in the health-care dollar, more of the diagnosis and therapy of the geriatric population will be held within the primary-care system. This book will help physicians with this task.

Even if the reader is in a system that makes specialty referral more readily available, we hope that the information provided herein will give him or her a greater ability to make the proper referral.

We have also tried to place more emphasis on the increased ability of orthopedic surgeons to provide not only more refined diagnosis for elderly patients but, using major advances in internal appliances, to operate on patients who would not have been candidates until recently. It is clear that although a multitude of nonsteroidal anti-inflammatory drugs have been introduced, their cumulative effect has not been as significant as the advances in total hip and total knee replacement over the past few decades.

Rheumatologists have also improved their diagnostic skills, and the increased emphasis on soft-tissue problems in the elderly has made the management of many musculoskeletal problems more rewarding for patients.

A review by Reynolds of data from the National Health Survey found that musculoskeletal disease was the most prevalent cause of chronic disability in the ambulatory population (2). In addition, it is estimated that approximately 175,000 patients, primarily elderly women, will suffer a hip fracture this year. Osteoarthrosis was mentioned 60 times per 1000 visits. It ranked third among women and seventh among men, pointing up the higher frequency of these disorders in women. In both sexes, there was a rising prevalence of rheumatic disorders after age 75, but, again, the most striking difference was among women, who experienced an almost twofold increase. It is no wonder that aspirin was fifth on the list of drugs used, with acetaminophen fourteenth and ibuprofen seventeenth. Analgesics were listed third in drugs ordered, after cardiac drugs and diuretics.

A general problem in dealing with elderly patients is the frequency with which they have multiple diseases. As a person ages, he or she becomes the heir of his or her lifetime events—for better or for worse. In old age, this heritage can mean an accumulation of diseases. A patient with arthritis may well have one of the health problems that exceed the frequency of osteoarthrosis in the elderly population: chronic ischemic heart disease, hypertension and diabetes. Such concurrent conditions may have only a minimal impact on the course or prognosis of the rheumatologic disease, and vice versa. In our experience in dealing with a geriatric group, we have noted the major interaction of these conditions to be on the drug therapy for the arthritis.

An example would be corticosteroids. We discuss in the text the beneficial effect of low-dose prednisone therapy for rheumatoid arthritis in elderly patients (3). We are all familiar with the side effect of fluid retention with corticosteroids.

Fluid retention may have deleterious effects on hypertension and on ischemic heart disease, particularly if there is any degree of cardiac failure. There is also the problem of gluconeogenesis, which would worsen diabetes mellitus. These side effects might be a major problem to a patient taking moderate to high doses of prednisone. Fortunately, there seems to be little deleterious effects with this drug at the lower dosages (an average of 5 mg of prednisone per day) that have a beneficial effect on an inflammatory arthritis. At this dosage, any fluid retention is minimal, and there is no appreciable change in the blood glucose level or need for increased use of glucose-lowering agents.

The important nonsteroidal anti-inflammatory drugs (NSAIDs) are the cyclo-oxygenase inhibitors. Major side effects can occur with these agents, including gastrointestinal problems, such as gastric irritation, microscopic to macroscopic bleeding, and ulcers.

Two mechanisms are responsible for these side effects. With the blockage of the cyclo-oxygenase enzyme, there is a reduction in the production of prostaglandin E. This prostaglandin is necessary to the maintenance of the mucin layer on the gastric mucosa. It is considered so necessary for this purpose that tests are under way with an NSAID that has prostaglandin E added to reverse this loss.

The other problem with NSAIDs is that they irritate the gastric mucosa while being absorbed through the stomach. The combination of these two side effects is more likely to go beyond the production of local bleeding to provoke the development of a gastric ulcer.

Gastroscopic studies (4) have demonstrated a reduction in the number and degree of irritative foci on the gastric mucosa when enteric-coated aspirin was compared to regular and buffered aspirin. There was no apparent difference in these effects between the regular aspirin and the aspirin with added antacid. It appears that we can limit direct irritation by preventing the material from being absorbed through the stomach. Hence, more enteric-coated, nonaspirin NSAIDS are becoming available.

It has been claimed that with some enteric coatings, the active constituent may not be absorbed. This was probably true when shellac coatings were used more than 20 years ago, but the new coatings will more reliably dissolve in the lower bowel. We have studied this aspect of NSAIDs in elderly patients (5) and have found no difference in the aspirin levels when patients took plain aspirin or enteric-coated aspirin for seven days.

The other drugs used in the management of musculoskeletal disease have their own problems, but because they are less widely used than the agents we have discussed, they will not be discussed at this point. The side effects of such agents are noted in various sections of this book.

ROBERT R. KARPMAN, M.D.
JOHN BAUM, M.D.

References

1. Koch, H., and Smith, M.C. Office-based ambulatory care for patients 75 years old and over. National Ambulatory Medical Care Survey 1980, 1981. Advance data from Vital and Health Statistics. No. 110 DHHS Pub. No. (PHS) 85–1250. Public Health Service, Hyattsville, MD., Aug. 21, 1985.
2. Reynolds, M.D. Prevalence of rheumatic diseases as causes of disability and complaints by ambulatory patients. *Arthritis Rheum.* 21:377–382, 1978.
3. Lockie, L.M., Gomez, E., and Smith, D.M. Low-dose adrenocorticosteroids in the management of rheumatoid arthritis. *Semin. Arthritis Rheum.* 12:373–381, 1983.
4. Lanza, F.L., Royer, G.L., Jr., and Nelson, R.S. Endoscopic evaluation of the effect of aspirin, buffered aspirin and enteric-coated aspirin on gastric and duodenal mucosa. *N. Engl. J. Med.* 303:136–138, 1980.
5. Orozco-Alcala, J.J., and Baum, J. Regular and enteric-coated aspirin: A re-evaluation. *Arthritis Rheum.* 22(9):1034–1037, 1979.

Contributors

David Haueisen, M.D.
Fellow
Arizona Hand Surgery Fellowship
Phoenix, Arizona

Franklin Kozin, M.D.
Member, Medical Group
Scripps Clinic and Research Foundation
La Jolla, California

Barry A. Kriegsfeld, M.D.
Neurosurgeon in Private Practice
Phoenix, Arizona

Lars-Goran Larsson, M.D.
Assistant Professor
Hospital for Rheumatic Diseases
Ostersund, Sweden

Carole Bernstein Lewis, Ph.D., R.P.T.
Adjunct Associate Professor
School of Allied Health Science
Department of Medicine
George Washington University
Washington, D.C.

L. Gregory Pawlson, M.D.
Associate Professor and Director of
Center for Aging Studies and Services
Department of Health Care
George Washington University
Washington, D.C.

Robert G. Volz, M.D.
Professor of Surgery
University of Arizona School of Medicine
Chief of Section of Orthopedic Surgery
University of Arizona
Tucson, Arizona

Robert Lee Wilson, M.D.
Chief of Hand Surgery Service
Maricopa Medical Center
Phoenix, Arizona
Associate in Surgery
University of Arizona
Tucson, Arizona

We wish to dedicate this book to our families whose patience and perseverance enabled us to complete this text. Special thanks goes to Kathleen Brill who was instrumental in typing and editing the multiple manuscripts.

Contents

AGING AND CLINICAL PRACTICE: MUSCULOSKELETAL DISORDERS

A Regional Approach

John Baum

Chapter 1

Arthritis and Rheumatism— An Overview

ETIOLOGY OF ARTHRITIS IN THE AGING

It is a truism that we all age and that the aging process produces changes. In the musculoskeletal system, a number of such changes lead to mild to severe disability. Among the elderly, the second most common affliction is osteoarthritis, surpassed in frequency only by cardiovascular disease. Osteoarthritis is usually regarded as a disease of old age, although it can develop relatively early in life as a result of trauma and similar conditions.

The changes seen in the cartilage of elderly people are considered manifestations of a degradative process. A number of theories have been proposed to explain why this process takes place. Table 1.1 lists some of them.

In this chapter, a detailed discussion of the various theories will not be given; however, some theories are of interest because they provide insights regarding measures that may have bearing on the prevention of osteoarthritis. Genetic variables can be altered only by selecting the proper parentage. However, the future may hold promise for modification of genetic makeup to improve resistance to disease, although financial and medical considerations may make this possibility unfeasible.

Nodes in the proximal interphalangeal joints (Bouchard's) and those in the terminal interphalangeal joints (Heberden's), have a strong familial pattern. Such nodes are encountered most often in female siblings and their daughters. These nodular changes can be acute, and the red, swollen, tender finger joints seen at presentation have led in some cases to a diagnosis of rheumatoid arthritis. In the most severe cases, the appearance is called ''jackstraw'' fingers, a term used by British physicians. The American term used to describe this condition is ''pick-up-sticks,'' referring to the lateral deviation of the fingers that causes them to overlap. This nodular condition can be distinguished clinically from rheumatoid arthritis, which mostly involves the metacarpophalangeal and proximal interphalangeal joints, usually sparing the distal joints. Acute cases eventually progress to a chronic state with the classical appearance of enlarged, nodular joints.

TABLE 1.1 Speculative Etiologic
Variables in the Aging of Cartilage

Genetic
Traumatic or mechanical stress
Immunologic variables
Enzymatic changes
The aging process—biochemical variables

Nonsteroidal anti-inflammatory drugs (NSAIDs) are usually prescribed. This author believes that patients over age 70 should not be started on full dosages, usually beginning treatment at half the recommended dosage. If there is no relief in about three weeks, the dosage can be increased. There appears to be an increased incidence of gastrointestinal side effects from NSAIDs in this age group. Peptic ulcer disease, in particular, may be aggravated by such drug therapy. A pure analgesic, such as acetaminophen or propoxyphene, in combination with an NSAID may provide greater relief in some cases.

In the author's experience, paraffin is helpful for patients with severe hand involvement. Paraffin is inexpensive and can be prepared easily in a double boiler. A physical therapist or an occupational therapist can teach a patient how to prepare and obtain benefit from a paraffin bath.

Joint trauma can begin with an injury early in life. Such an injury produces incongruity of the joint, which results in abnormal stress on the joint surfaces. The changes that occur are similar to those seen in degenerative joint disease. It is clear that the wear and pathologic change are more apparent where the bones are close together or where the fit causes undue stress on an area of cartilage.

Immunologic variables have long been considered a possible etiologic basis for degenerative joint disease. Cooke (1), an orthopedic surgeon and immunologist, has studied cartilage removed surgically from patients with osteoarthritis. Below the surface of the cartilage, he found evidence of immune complexes, as revealed by immunofluorescent staining of deposits of immunoglobulins and complement. It is believed that deposition occurs as synovial fluid is pushed into cartilage by the force of activity. This mechanism is the normal means of nutrition for this tissue. Proteins, including immune complexes, can also travel relatively deeply into cartilage. With joint motion, there is back and forth flow, and proteins can return to the synovial fluid. Immune complexes in synovial fluid can activate complement and produce other effects of inflammation.

Inflammation result in the release of enzymes from invading macrophages, polymorphonuclear leukocytes and stimulated cells of the pannus. Proteases, elastases, collagenases and other enzymes are released into synovial fluid and attack any materials bathed by the fluid. In such a disease as rheumatoid arthritis, in which there is maximal inflammatory activity, large amounts of these enzymes are present; however, when there is minimal inflammatory activity, as in degenerative joint disease, the concentrations of these enzymes are low. The white cell count in the fluid gives a rough estimate of enzyme concentrations and resultant damage. However, the enzymatic activity responsible for fibrillation of cartilage, a hallmark of the degeneration seen in the aging process, has yet to be precisely determined. Whether enzymatic activity is, in fact, the mechanism of the breakdown has not been proved.

A variety of biochemical changes in the joints may be a result of the aging process. Fibrillation of cartilage may be due to such biochemical effects. By changing its composition, the concentration of chondroitin sulfate decreases markedly during the aging process. By contrast, the concentration of another component of cartilage, keratin sulfate, is initially low but increases with age. The enzymes found in later life constitute a different group, although some of them are the same as those whose concentrations increase during inflammation. They include proteases, collagenases, hyaluronidases and mucopolysaccharidases.

In addition to enzymatic changes, there may be increases in the water content of cartilage, a biophysical change of the aging process.

The specifics of degenerative joint disease will be covered in other chapters. This disease mostly afflicts the elderly. Studies from around the world have shown that the incidence of degenerative joint disease begins to accelerate at about age 60 (2).

A study conducted in Tecumseh, Michigan, revealed that 30 percent of the women could be diagnosed as having osteoarthritis on the basis of their clinical history; however, only about 15 percent of the men had such a history. The proportions increased after physical examination to approximately 40 and 20 percent, respectively. This type of population survey provides the most reliable information about the prevalence of a disease. The history and physical examination are better than roentgenographic surveys, which might demonstrate osteoarthritic changes but do not necessarily correlate with clinical complaints.

Degenerative joint disease is typically managed with an NSAID. Although it has been pointed out that this disease is accompanied by minimal inflammation, even such minimal activity mandates the use of an NSAID. Moreover, it is advisable to use an enteric-coated NSAID because such preparations reportedly help protect the gastric mucosa (3). For patients who continue to suffer pain, addition of a pure analgesic agent, such as acetaminophen or propoxyphene, will provide greater relief. Physical methods are also helpful. Application of heat produces muscle relaxation, whereas application of cold produces analgesia and thus permits increased activity. The therapist determines which modality best suits a patient. Increasing muscle strength should be the aim of physical therapy. An overall increase in strength relieves some of the stress on the affected joints.

Secondary osteoarthritis is also encountered in the elderly. A traumatic basis is easiest to recognize from the history and occasionally from the physical examination. Rheumatoid arthritis destroys cartilage and bone and thereby leads eventually to degenerative changes. Chondrocalcinosis with repeated episodes of joint inflammation caused by the irritative effect of calcium pyrophosphate crystals leads to degenerative joint disease that is difficult to distinguish from the primary type. McCarty has described six patterns of chondrocalcinosis (4). The most frequent form, pseudogout, presents as acute, gouty-like attacks. The three types that appear similar to osteoarthritis can mimic this form or be manifested by occasional acute attacks. A fifth type of chondrocalcinosis can be demonstrated only roentgenographically. In the last form, the disease has an appearance similar to that of rheumatoid arthritis. In some patients, roentgeno-graphic studies have demonstrated rheumatoid arthritis secondary to chondrocalci-nosis, and clinical differentiation from primary rheumatoid arthritis of unknown origin is difficult in such cases (5).

Rheumatoid arthritis has a variable presentation in the elderly. It may be of acute onset, the classical presentation in such cases consisting of acute swelling and tenderness of several joints in a symmetric pattern. The metacarpophalangeal joints and wrists are often involved, as they are in young patients. Elderly patients who have suffered from degenerative joint disease have other complaints. They describe morning stiffness lasting up to several hours and involvement of additional joints with more severe swelling and pain. Although it may seem that a new disease is developing, physicians should be mindful of this often misdiagnosed variant of rheumatoid arthritis in the elderly. Studies of joint fluid are helpful in this regard, particularly in elderly patients, because they may reveal some other cause of the acute inflammation. Characteristically, the joint fluid has an inflammatory aspect, showing a high white cell count and a shift to mostly polymorphonuclear leukocytes. Studies of the peripheral blood show an increased erythrocyte sedimentation rate and, in many cases, rheumatoid factor is seen.

An epidemiology group in Sweden recently found that in 20 percent of patients age 79, the onset of rheumatoid arthritis occurred after age 75 (7).

The poor predictive value of some tests and procedures usually used to help or confirm this diagnosis was disappointing. Roentgenographic studies had only a 50 percent predictive value for morning stiffness and 25 percent for rheumatoid factor. These figures again point out the importance of the history and physical examination. Although roentgenographic studies are usually thought of in light of their ability to demonstrate disease characteristics (e.g., erosion), interestingly enough, the roentgenographic appearance had a higher predictive value (65 percent) for osteoarthritis of the finger joints and wrists. The patient population in the Swedish study was too small (three men and three women) to establish any sex-related differences for the disease.

The disease in elderly patients can be as intense as that seen in young patients. Treatment starts with an NSAID with the understanding that relatively low dosages should be the rule in patients age 70 or older. If a patient does not respond to this treatment, a long-acting agent should be added. A gold compound is typically chosen. Standard therapy has long consisted of an intramuscular compound, such as gold sodium thiomalate, but the recent availability of oral gold has made administration easier and reduced toxicity, although such gold compounds may be less effective. A major side effect of gold compounds is loosening of the bowels, which may be in some elderly patients who suffer from constipation. These compounds do not appear to be more toxic to the bone marrow and kidney in elderly patients.

It is in this group that the recommendation made by Lockie and associates (6) to use low dosages of prednisone is of benefit. In the author's experience, prednisone in combination with an NSAID is often more effective. Lockie and associates used a dosage of 5 mg per day. The author usually starts at or below this dosage. Prednisone is used in patients who are not responding well to therapy. It is occasionally added when a patient has not responded well to therapy and there is reason not to wait until the long-acting agent has been demonstrated to be effective. Starting with 1 mg tablets enables the author to find a low but beneficial dosage. Prednisone reduces the period of morning stiffness and decreases the inflammation. If morning stiffness is the major problem, the drug is often most effective when taken at night.

Gout has changed in frequency in modern times. Although it is regarded as a prime example of a hereditary disease, there is a strong interplay of environmental variables. When its onset is in the early decades of life, it continues to be a disease of males. A characteristic amusingly portrayed in eighteenth-century prints was the frequency and appearance of the disease in the upper socioeconomic strata of society. Most often, gout was correctly considered to be the product of the diet of the times, excessively loaded with high-purine foods and wine, principally port. A high-purine diet of meat and game (e.g., pheasant) is a well-known cause of hyperuricemia. However, it is not as well known that because of the shipping practices for this wine from Portugal, it is heavily contaminated with lead. The latter material causes retention of uric acid and when it is the only etiologic factor gives rise to a typical elevation of the uric acid concentration and acute gouty attacks, producing what is known as saturnine gout. Saturn was the alchemists' sign for lead. In modern times, lead has been a major contaminant of "moonshine" whiskey. In recent years, the author identified this disease in a man from the Deep South who maintained a taste for (and had a supplier of) this brew.

In northern Europe, the major cause of hyperuricemia, and thus a frequent causative agent, is the use of diuretic drugs. In the Swedish study cited previously, hyperuricemia was found in 16 percent of cases. A hereditary basis was thought to be responsible in 5 percent, the remainder being due to drug usage. However, the prevalence of gouty arthritis was only 1.3 percent. The investigators stated that "diseases causing hyperuricemia are of more importance in the elderly than in lower age groups." It is clear from the figures presented that hyperuricemia in the elderly does not require management because the prevalence of gout is much lower than the prevalence of increased serum levels of uric acid. Moderate cases of hyperuricemia do not warrant management, which should be reserved for cases of gout.

Another cause of hyperuricemia in the elderly is chronic myeloproliferative disease (8). This condition usually starts in later life. Yu and colleagues reported that the blood disorder started between ages 50 and 59 in most of a series of patients, with secondary gout starting about seven years later. Secondary gout included polycythemia vera, myeloid metaplasia and chronic leukemia. It appears that in such cases, the long duration of the elevated level of uric acid leads to the development of arthritis. This problem is no longer prevalent because most physicians recognize secondary hyperuricemia and use such drugs as allopurinol to control the level of uric acid.

There is still debate over when and how to manage hyperuricemia. When it was realized that diuretics, particularly thiazides, could precipitate gout in elderly patients, a uricosemic agent was added if the diuretic had to be continued. If the level of uric acid was not excessive, the patients condition could be monitored, and if a problem arose (i.e., acute arthritis), treatment would be instituted. From the data in the Swedish study, it is also clear that gout does not develop in all patients with hyperuricemia. The author believes that if the level is not excessively high, the patient should not be treated. Determining the concentration of uric acid at regular intervals allows control of the situation.

An acute gouty attack is traditionally managed with colchicine. Standard practice is to give 0.5 mg at hourly intervals until 7 mg has been given or until the acute attack responds or diarrhea develops. To avoid diarrhea, which can be devastating in an elderly patient, colchicine can be given intravenously. One or two vials (2 mg) can be injected well diluted and with care because colchicine can cause severe damage to tissue if the vial leaks. If the physician is aware of the diagnosis from knowledge that hyperuricemia exists or on the basis of an aspirate from the joint that shows crystals in the synovial fluid, administration of an NSAID is preferable. Such agents do not act as quickly as intravenous colchicine but do not cause diarrhea. A loading dose should be followed by high doses in the first 24 hours. For example, with phenylbutazone, the initial dose is 150 to 200 mg, followed by enough doses in the next 24 hours to give a total dosage of 600 to 800 mg. With indomethacin, the initial dose is 50 mg, followed by 200 mg over the next 24 hours. Drug therapy should be conducted at maintenance levels over the next four to five days.

It may be difficult to achieve a low serum level of uric acid in elderly patients receiving a uricosuric agent, such as probenecid. Such patients should maintain a high fluid intake (the standard recommendation is about 3 liters daily) as well as alkalinization of the urine. The xanthine oxidase inhibitor allopurinol is easier to use in elderly patients because these recommendations do not have to be followed.

The differential diagnosis of arthritis can be diagrammed by use of an algorithm that will aid in determining the cause of joint or back pain in a patient over age 60 who presents to a primary-care physician. Because the algorithm is only an aid in making the diagnosis, the reader should note that arbitrary levels rather than ranges have been used in relation to various laboratory tests. The values shown in the algorithm are those that are applicable in the laboratories used by the author; the reader may adjust them according to personal judgment. The erythrocyte sedimentation rate was determined by the Westergren method. It is advisable to use this technique because the value so obtained is more likely to be abnormal in cases of inflammation than it would be if Wintrobe and Landsberg's method were used. In elderly patients, in whom the value may be lower for a number of reasons, the difference between the two tests may be substantial. The values for rheumatoid factor are those considered abnormal by the latex agglutination test in most laboratories.

A polarizing microscope and a special red filter are required for distinguishing between uric acid crystals and calcium pyrophosphate crystals in synovial fluid. If a regular light microscope is available, Polaroid filters in the form of sheets can be used. One is placed over the eyepiece and one over the condenser. By rotating the filters, the light is polarized and the crystals can be visualized. Joint fluid can be held in a refrigerator overnight and sent to a laboratory for evaluation the next morning if the physician is doing the aspiration in his or her office.

If a patient presents with joint pain, the physician must take a history and do a physical examination to establish the presence of arthritis. Pain by itself is arthralgia and may reflect only a soft-tissue problem. Such complaints will be discussed later because they are frequently encountered in the elderly. If there is warmth, tenderness and, especially, swelling, a diagnosis of arthritis is likely. A complaint of back pain is more difficult to assess. These findings are rarely associated with arthritis. As with the hips, the skeletal structures are too far from the surface to show inflammatory changes.

The history sometimes includes complaints arising from other chronic problems. Swelling of the ankles secondary to congestive heart failure can obscure primary arthritis. Conversely, swelling of the ankles secondary to a rheumatic condition may be misinterpreted as resulting from heart failure. The dates of the onsets of signs and symptoms can sometimes be forgotten because of a failing memory.

The author tries to make a single diagnosis correspond with a patient's signs and symptoms. Again, it should be remembered that a disease starting in old age is often superimposed on some underlying disease of long duration, a disease that began before the arthritic complaints started. This is true for the rheumatic diseases. For example, it must be realized that degenerative joint disease does not preclude the onset of rheumatoid arthritis in old age, but it does make the diagnosis difficult. Recognizable changes in a patient's signs and symptoms are most helpful clinically. A patient who has had degenerative joint disease but who now complains of prolonged morning stiffness and increasing fatigue should undergo a workup to determine whether rheumatoid arthritis is the cause.

If arthritis has been clearly diagnosed, it should be characterized as monarticular or polyarticular. Monarticular disease is most often seen in the knee. Polyarticular disease is more the rule in this age group, although conditions usually thought of as monarticular, such as gout, can occur in several joints.

Algorithm

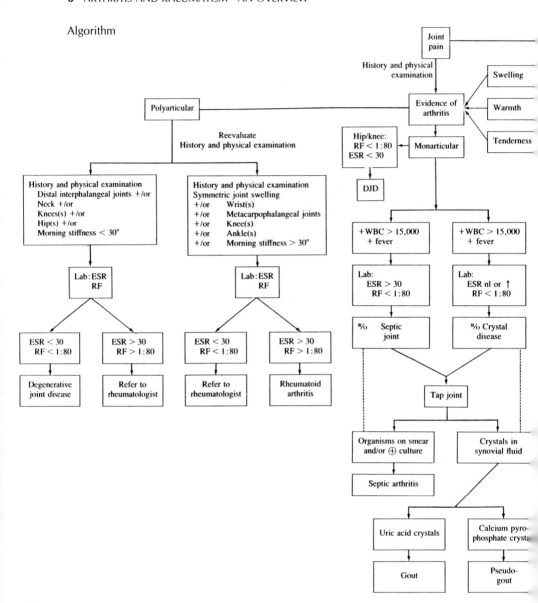

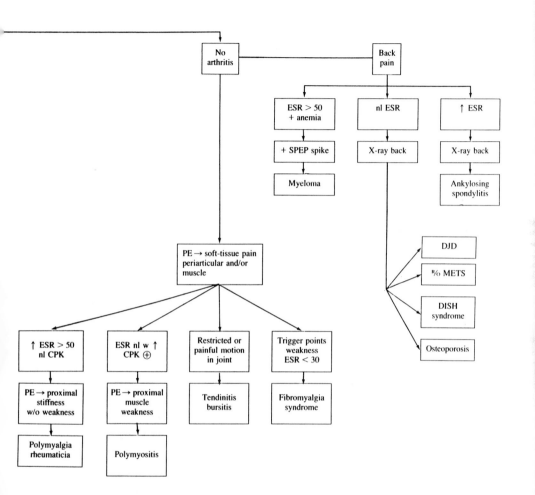

If the disease in an elderly patient is polyarticular, the physical examination is especially informative. Elderly patients may have nodes in the proximal interphalangeal joints (Bouchard's) and in the terminal interphalangeal joints (Heberden's) of the hands. The most distinctive characteristic of rheumatoid arthritis is that it involves the metacarpophalangeal joints, particularly the second and third ones. Wrist involvement is frequent in rheumatoid arthritis but must be differentiated on the basis of the physical examination from involvement of the first carpometacarpal joint (base of the thumb). Patients with degenerative joint disease describe wrist pain when only this joint is involved. Swelling and warmth of the wrist with restriction of flexion and extension are usually indicative of inflammatory disease. Ankle involvement is an unusual finding in degenerative joint disease but is commonly seen in rheumatoid arthritis.

Laboratory tests help support the evidence collected from the history and physical examination. Extensive tests may be needed, especially if the diagnosis is in doubt. However, relatively few tests are required in an elderly patient if the clinician has a working diagnosis. This algorithm indicates the need for only an erythrocyte sedimentation rate and a test for rheumatoid factor. The results of these laboratory studies must be interpreted with care because both tests can be positive in elderly patients.

A low titer of rheumatoid factor (below the normal range in a given laboratory) is of little help. By contrast, a high titer is not diagnostic but helps confirm the clinical findings. The same is true of the erythrocyte sedimentation rate, which increases with age so that only a higher than expected rise is diagnostically helpful. This point is a subject of controversy, however. Recent studies performed by the author and a colleague (unpublished observations) did not demonstrate a rise in the sedimentation rate with age. The best data on this change with age have been reported by Bottiger and Svedberg (9), who studied a large patient population.

In that study, the upper end of the normal range was 20 mm per hour in men over age 50 and 30 mm in women of the same age. On the basis of this information, a rate of 40 mm per hour or higher in a man or 50 mm or higher in a woman over age 50 should be considered highly suspicious of inflammatory activity if degenerative joint disease has been previously diagnosed. Nonetheless, a number of nonrheumatic inflammatory diseases are associated with an elevated sedimentation rate. For this reason, lower values are used here so that they may be correlated with the clinical data.

Even though roentgenographic studies may be helpful, they have not been included because radiographic changes seen in the diseases addressed by this algorithm may not be apparent in the early stages. A roentgenogram may demonstrate the classical changes of degenerative joint disease. If rheumatoid arthritis coexists, erosive destruction of the articular surface may not be apparent until the disease has progressed considerably. If the disease is also accompanied by chondrocalcinosis, the diagnosis may become more confusing. Although the clinical diagnosis may be degenerative joint disease alone, some patients present with severe joint involvement that mimics gout (pseudogout) and even inflammation of a number of joints that suggests rheumatoid arthritis. If none of the various diseases in the algorithm is the diagnosis, a more detailed workup is required.

If a patient with pain does not have peripheral joint arthritis, the investigation follows another path. Back pain often cannot be ascribed to arthritis on the basis of the presenting complaints. Like the joints of the hips, the joints of the back are so deeply buried that a complaint of pain cannot be ascribed to inflammatory disease.

The algorithm shows that the erythrocyte sedimentation rate helps determine the path the investigation will now take. A substantial elevation of the rate in combination with anemia points to the diagnosis. In such cases, if serum immunoelectrophoresis shows a spike in the globulin area, multiple myeloma is the likely diagnosis. Myeloma may be associated with only minimal osteoporosis. If the clinician had relied solely on a roentgenogram to make the diagnosis, this condition could not be distinguished from primary osteoporosis in most cases. If invasion of the vertebral bodies is severe, pathologic fractures with collapse of the vertebral bodies will be seen in many cases. Laboratory studies confirm the diagnosis.

Roentgenography in degenerative joint disease shows characteristic changes. In the back, the osteophytes of the vertebral bodies are visualized. There is also narrowing of the spaces between the bodies. Ankylosis is a rare finding. The clinical manifestations bear little resemblance to the severity of the roentgenographic findings.

Another condition that can be diagnosed at this point but only with knowledge of its roentgenographic appearance is diffuse idiopathic skeletal hyperostosis (Forestier's disease). This disease is manifested by calcium deposits in the ligaments of the anterior and right lateral margins of the thoracic vertebrae. Deposits are seen on both sides of the lumbar vertebrae. It is generally accepted that the asymmetric pattern in the thoracic area is due to the pulsations of the thoracic aorta, which prevent formation of deposits on that side. Deposits are also seen in the cervical vertebrae and at peripheral sites of insertion of tendons and ligaments. Another feature is the tendency of the calcium deposits to appear to curve downward, unlike the osteophytes seen in degenerative joint disease, which have a lateral pattern of growth.

Forestier's disease is mostly an affliction of the elderly, being rarely reported before age 50. It is virtually impossible to diagnose without roentgenographic studies because nothing in the history or physical examination is pathognomonic. Back pain, the most frequent symptom, is similar to that seen with degenerative joint disease. Restriction of back motion, which might be expected, has not been described. An association with hypertension and stroke has been reported but has yet to be explained. It has also been claimed that there is an association with diabetes, but this report has not been confirmed.

If the erythrocyte sedimentation rate is moderately elevated and the patient has a stiff back, the investigation focuses on the possibility of ankylosing spondylitis. This inflammatory disorder is mostly seen in young men, in whom the disease eventually progresses to the full-blown syndrome. Ankylosing spondylitis is characterized by stiffness of the back and, in many cases, involvement of the hip joints. The disease begins at advanced age in rare cases. It is usually not a likely possibility in the differential diagnosis in an elderly patient.

Carcinoma metastasizing to the spine can cause back pain. Some tumors are accompanied by osteoporosis alone, whereas others with extensive involvement cause the vertebral bodies to collapse. The erythrocyte sedimentation rate is elevated more often with metastatic disease than with uncomplicated cancer.

In patients with arthritis of the knee, the differential diagnosis is increasingly including the possibility of Lyme disease as reports of cases in the United States continue to accumulate (10). The disease has been reported in 14 states, primarily in the Northeast, Midwest and West and has been described in patients as old as 77 (11).

The presenting skin lesion is erythema chronicum migrans, which may be accompanied by flulike or meningitis-like symptoms. The diagnosis relies on a high index of suspicion. Clues to the diagnosis are whether the patient in an endemic area, being exposed in the woods or brush, and whether he or she had the typical prodomata of the arthritis (e.g., rash, fever, headache and malaise). Serologic tests demonstrate antibodies to the causative spirochete in less than 50 percent of cases.

The arthritis should be managed with high doses of penicillin. Intravenous administration may be required if oral therapy is unsuccessful. In chronic cases, synovectomy is occasionally necessary.

Interestingly enough, many patients describe joint pain but do not show evidence of arthritis on physical examination. Such patients may have one of the conditions that fall under the rubric of soft-tissue rheumatism.

Several diseases create muscle and joint problems but are not accompanied by evidence of joint disease. Muscle weakness and stiffness are the predominant complaints. A marked elevation of the erythrocyte sedimentation rate (greater than 50 mm per hour) points to a diagnosis of polymyalgia rheumatica in such cases. Few other conditions cause such an elevation in patients with the major complaints of muscle weakness and stiffness. Laboratory studies of creatinine phosphokinase show a normal level of this muscle enzyme.

Elderly patients with polymyalgia rheumatica have severe morning stiffness, mostly of the hips and shoulder girdle. They have to swing their legs over the edge of the bed and then rock the upper part of their bodies to stand upright and move away from the bed. This stiffness is considered more bothersome than any muscle or joint pain they may report. Therapy with an NSAID is usually of little help. On the other hand, therapy with a corticosteroid confirms the diagnosis, as evidenced by a dramatic response to a low dosage of prednisone (10 to 15 mg per day). Prednisone provides marked relief of the stiffness—so much so that patients claim to feel normal in one or two days.

Temporal arteritis is known to be associated with polymyalgia rheumatica, developing in about 15 percent of cases. Although some physicians recommend biopsy of the temporal artery in all patients with polymyalgia rheumatica, the author orders a biopsy only if the history or physical examination suggests arteritis. Evidence of this possibility includes transient episodes of loss of vision, headache, constitutional symptoms (fever and weight loss) or tenderness or swelling of the temporal artery. If arteritis is documented, high doses of corticosteroids are required for a successful outcome.

Another muscle disease seen in the elderly is dermatomyositis (polymyositis when unaccompanied by a rash). An epidemiologic study (12) has shown that the incidence of the disease is highest between ages 45 and 54 and that the frequency is significantly higher in blacks, particularly women between the ages of 55 and 64.

The rash is characterized by a purple discoloration of the upper eyelids. There may also be an erythematous rash on the face, arms and trunk. The rash may be pruritic with induration and edema of the subcutaneous tissues. Patients describe progressive weakness of the proximal muscles, more severe than the weakness seen in polymyalgia rheumatica.

The erythrocyte sedimentation rate is elevated or normal. The diagnosis can be confirmed by electromyography or biopsy of the affected muscles.

The most important feature of this syndrome in elderly patients is its relationship to malignant lesions. A number of review articles have documented that such an association exists, one report describing it in 15 percent of cases (13). The malignant lesion preceded or followed the myositis by up to two years. In some cases, identification and removal of the lesion result in resolution of the myositis.

Management usually involves a course of corticosteroids, but a high dosage is often required. The dosage and duration of therapy required for a successful outcome, however, often cause side effects.

In the author's experience, the most common soft-tissue problems are mild, benign lesions. Of 600 clinic referrals, 108 (17.8 percent) were diagnosed as soft-tissue rheumatism (14). In no case was there evidence of generalized inflammation that would provoke an elevation of the erythrocyte sedimentation rate.

A form of nonarticular rheumatism that is especially common in elderly patients is bursitis. A bursa reduces the friction where tendons or muscles move over one another or cross in opposite directions. Some bursae cushion bony prominences. There are more than 150 bursae in the body. Some are present throughout life, and some form during life as the need arises. It is clear that if one lives long enough, the stress of daily functioning will lead to the development of bursitis as continued use or strain occurs.

Among the most common types of bursitis are subdeltoid, trochanteric and pes anserinus. The subdeltoid bursa is frequently the origin of shoulder pain in adults. Patients with subdeltoid bursitis experience limitation of motion, particularly when trying to raise the hand to the head. They are occasionally awakened at night when they roll over on the affected shoulder.

Physical examination reveals tenderness with pressure laterally just below the acromion but little or no pain when the shoulder is palpated anteriorly. Such patients have a "painful arc." There is little or no pain when the arm is passively raised until its angle is about 30 degrees; the pain persists for the next 60 degrees and disappears at that point as the humerus rotates from under the acromion, thus relieving the pressure on the bursa. The diagnosis can be rapidly confirmed within minutes after instilling some lidocaine into the bursa. The author usually gives 1 or 2 ml of a depo-steroid after the analgesic agent.

Patients with trochanteric bursitis suffer from hip pain and state that they cannot lie on the affected side at night because the pain is so severe. True hip pain usually presents as pain in the groin and not in a lateral location, as encountered in patients with trochanteric bursitis.

Physical examination demonstrates a normal range of hip motion but frequently reveals moderate to marked tenderness with pressure over the greatest trochanter. Instillation of lidocaine over the most tender area affords almost instantaneous relief. A long-acting depo-steroid can be given after the lidocaine.

The most interesting bursitis is the pes anserinus variety (15). This form is especially common in overweight elderly women referred with osteoarthritis of the knee that has not responded to any NSAID. The knee pain is usually unilateral but may be bilateral. Pain is experienced when climbing stairs, when getting up after prolonged sitting and when bending the knee. Many patients report that they cannot lie on their sides at night because the pressure of one knee on the other is painful and wakes them up.

Physical examination demonstrates a normal range of knee motion with little or no pain. Crepitus is reported in some cases. There is little or no pain with pressure over the joint margin but severe pain with only moderate pressure over the pes anserinus, which is located medially about two inches below the joint margin.

Although this condition is being considered a form of bursitis, there is evidence that it may be tendinitis at the point of insertion of a muscle in that area, the sartorius, gracilis or semitendinosus.

Lidocaine injected directly into the affected area affords almost instantaneous relief. Because patients report a long-lasting effect (from days to years) with this local anesthetic, a depo-steroid is reserved for refractory cases to protect the integrity of the tendons.

The last soft-tissue rheumatism presented in the algorithm is fibromyalgia, or fibrositis. The author prefers to use the former term because inflammation has not been clearly identified in this syndrome. Some well-defined signs and symptoms can be used to characterize this condition. It is a chronic problem characterized by "trigger points" in certain restricted areas, mostly around the shoulders, back and pelvis. The pain (most often around the shoulders) may not be constant and is usually exacerbated by cold, dampness or tension. Patients sleep poorly, often awakening during the night and waking up the next morning with typical discomfort. The pain can be relieved temporarily by taking a hot shower. Frequent bouts of fatigue are common during the day.

Physical examination demonstrates the trigger points, tender areas from which pain radiates, for example, from spots on the posterior aspect of the deltoid muscle to the neck or down the arm. The erythrocyte sedimentation rate is normal, and other laboratory tests are not informative.

Lidocaine injected into the trigger points relieves the pain. The author does not use depo-steroids because the lidocaine usually has a long-lasting effect. The sleep problem is helped with a single night-time dose of a tricyclic antidepressant. It is not clear whether the effect of such agents is from their antidepressant activity or whether they have a beneficial effect on nonrapid eye movement (stage 4) sleep.

This simple algorithm takes into account most musculoskeletal diseases encountered in elderly patients.

In this chapter, reference has been made to the use of NSAIDs as well as corticosteroids. In any elderly patient, the watchword is caution in the use of any drug. The aging process alters the way in which drugs are metabolized. Most NSAIDs are metabolized by the liver and excreted by the kidneys. Elderly patients may have a number of diseases involving these organs and thus affecting the way drugs used to manage such diseases are handled. For this reason, the breakdown and excretion of drugs used to manage rheumatic diseases are altered. In the management of rheumatoid arthritis and degenerative joint disease, for example, it is generally safer to start with half the recommended dosage of an NSAID in a patient over age 70. If the medication is not effective after about three weeks, the dosage can be increased.

REFERENCES

1. Cooke, T.D., Bennet, E.L., and Ohro, O. Identification of immunoglobulins and complement components in articular collagenous tissues of patients with idiopathic osteoarthritis, in Nuki, G. (ed.): *The Actiopathogenesis of Osteoarthritis.* Pitman, Tunbridge Wells, England, 1980, pp. 144–155.
2. Mikkelsen, W.M., Dodge, H.J., Duff, I.F., and Kato, H. Estimates of the prevalence of rheumatic diseases in the population of Tecumseh, Michigan, 1959–1960. *J. Chronic Dis.* 20:369, 1967.
3. Lanza, F.L., Royes, G.L., Jr., and Nelson, R.D. Endoscopic evaluation of the effects of aspirin, buffered aspirin and enteric-coated aspirin on gastric and duodenal mucosa. *N. Engl. J. Med.* 303:136–138, 1980.
4. McCarty D. Pathogenesis and treatment of crystal-induced inflammation, in McCarty D. (ed.): *Arthritis and allied conditions,* ed 9. Lea and Febiger, 1979, pp. 1245–1254.
5. Castillo, E., and Calderon, J. Roentgenographic features of the arthropathy associated with CPPD crystal deposition disease. A comparative study with primary osteoarthritis. *J. Rheum.* 12:1154–1158, 1985.

6. Lockie, L.M., Gomez E., and Smith, D.M. Low-dose adreyoeorticosteroids in the management of rheumatoid arthritis. *Semin. Arthritis Rheum.* 12:373–381, 1983.
7. Bergstrom, G., Bjelle, A., Sorensen, L.B., Sundh, V., and Svanborg, A. Prevalence of rheumatoid arthritis, osteoarthritis, chondrocalcinosis and gouty arthritis at age 79. *J. Rheum.* 13:527–534, 1986.
8. Yu, T., Weinreb, N., Wittman, R., and Wasserman, L.A. Secondary gout associated with myeloproliferative disorders. *Semin. Arthritis Rheum.* 5:247–256, 1976
9. Bottinger, L.E., and Svedberg, C.A. Normal erythrocyte sedimentation rate and age. *Brit. Med. J.* 2:85–87, 1967.
10. Schmid, G.P., Horsley, R., Steere, A.C., Hanrahan, J.P., Davis, J.P., Bowen, G.S., Osterhold, M.T., Weisfeld, J.S., Hightower, A.W., and Broome, C.V. Surveillance of Lyme Disease in the United States, 1982. *J. Infect. Dis.* 151:1144–1149, 1985.
11. Shresta, M., Grodzicki, R.L., and Steere, A.C. Diagnosing early lyme disease. *Amer. J. Med.* 78:235–240, 1985.
12. Medsger, T.A., Dawson, W.N., and Masi, A.T. The epidemiology of dermatomyositis. *Amer. J. Med.* 48:715–723, 1970.
13. Barnes, B.E. Dermatomyositis and malignancy: A review of the literature. *Ann. Intern. Med.* 84:68–76, 1976.
14. Larsson, L-G., and Baum, J. Non-articular rheumatism in an aging population. *Clin. Rheum. Pract.* 4:15–19, 1986.
15. Larsson, L-G., and Baum, J. The syndrome of anserina bursitis: An overlooked diagnosis. *Arthritis Rheum.* 28:1062–1065, 1985.

Barry A. Kriegsfeld
John Baum

Chapter 2

Neck and Back

DISORDERS OF THE NECK

Back pain (including neck pain) is a major public-health problem. Data from England show that about 80 percent of the population may have back pain at some time, and Jayson from Manchester has stated that "the magnitude of the back pain problem is daunting" (1).

This condition is so ubiquitous that a patient with back pain is sometimes viewed as a "back" by the physician, who neglects to investigate for any of the numerous causes of such complaints. Although most pain in the axial skeleton is *low*-back pain, the spine stretches from the cervical portion to the coccyx, and any segment can be involved. We will start from the top with problems of the cervical spine.

Neck pain can be as confusing to geriatricians as back pain. Like low-back pain, neck pain requires a careful history and physical examination. Important clues are found in a patient's description of the pain, the distribution and radiation of the symptoms and exacerbating factors.

Some forms of neck pain due to trauma and stress span the decades. For example, young patients often have a history of trauma. "Whiplash" caused by a motor vehicle accident is a classical injury of this type. In this patient group, sports injuries can also produce this lesion, which is caused by acute cervical strain.

The differential diagnosis in young and middle-aged patients includes psychologic stress, which can result in neck and head pain. This type of stress is a pure soft-tissue problem that is unaccompanied by skeletal changes or abnormalities. However, such changes later dominate the picture. Thus, in middle-aged and elderly patients, pain in the cervical spine is often and properly ascribed to degenerative joint disease. In some cases, a major complaint is "crackling" in the neck.

Although it is widely believed that whiplash involves the cervical vertebrae almost exclusively, such injuries reflect damage to the soft tissue of the cervical spine. Before cervical restraints were standard automobile equipment, this type of injury was more common. The lesion is produced when a rear-end collision results in rapid acceleration. The victim's head moves backward rapidly (particularly if no restraint is present), causing hyperextension of the neck. This movement of the head is followed by forward motion, a compensatory hyperflexion. Each movement leads to a different type of injury. Hyperextension is any angle greater than 45 degrees, the normal limit. Hyperextension mainly affects the soft tissues in the anterior part of the neck, usually around the level of the lower cervical vertebrae. The major damage is to the anterior longitudinal ligament, which is torn by the stress. The subsequent forward rebound produces relative hyperflexion, relative because forward movement is restricted by the chin striking the chest. However, the force is often strong enough to tear the nuchal ligament.

Signs and symptoms are not always evident immediately, sometimes not appearing for 24 to 48 hours. Clinical manifestations that appear immediately may consist of pain referred to the shoulders, back of the head or arms. Pain referred down the arms can reflect more serious damage, such as displacement of a disk causing compression of a nerve root. If vascular damage has occurred, other manifestations will be encountered, depending on the vessel involved. Bleeding with a tear of the anterior longitudinal ligament may produce a retropharyngeal hematoma, causing dysphagia. Damage to the vertebrobasilar artery is said to be a cause of tinnitus, whereas spasm of the vertebral artery is a cause of vertigo. These problems are almost always managed by an orthopedist or a neurosurgeon and are almost always more serious in elderly than in young patients.

Although severe osteoarthritis of the cervical spine can produce local signs and symptoms, it is more likely to cause referred pain. Compere has stated that "pain in the shoulder radiating down the arm to the elbow or into the hand and fingers is *nearly always due to a cervical lesion,* since primary lesions of the shoulder usually do not produce radiating pain beyond the elbow" (2). Pain localized to the neck is usually reported by elderly patients, who also sometimes describe crepitus in the neck with movement. Occasionally, the crepitus can be felt if the fingers are placed on the spinous processes and the patient is asked to reproduce the motions that induce the crepitus. There is no relationship of crepitus to any clinical syndrome. A tumor of the cervical spine is more likely to produce pain in the shoulder and arm.

Fibromyalgia is an underdiagnosed cause of neck pain. The trigger points in this condition are mostly spread around the paraspinal and deltoid muscles. The author has seen many patients with neck pain who had definite trigger points at the angle of the neck and shoulder with radiation into the neck. Relief of the pain after injection of the trigger points with lidocaine helped confirm the diagnosis.

Cervical radiculopathies other than those related to rheumatoid arthritis are relatively rare in the elderly. In a few cases, severe hypertrophic osteoarthritis narrows the involved vertebral foramen so much that an exiting nerve root becomes compressed (Figure 2.1c). The distribution of the pain depends on which nerve root is involved, and the pain is usually followed by a loss of motor and sensory function as well as by reflex changes. In severe cases, surgical decompression is required. A conservative regimen of bedrest, an analgesic and physical therapy is usually helpful. Surgical traction, other than relieving muscle spasm, does not appear to be helpful in decompressing an involved nerve root.

Patients with hypertrophic osteoarthritis or Forestier's disease may suffer from dysphagia, caused by compression of the esophagus by a large anterior bone spur. If the dysphagia is severe, the spur may have to be removed (Figure 2.1b).

The most definitive lesion of the cervical spine is found in rheumatoid arthritis. It consists of osteoporosis, erosion and narrowing of the disks (3). In addition, instability of the atlantoaxial and subaxial joints occurs in severe cases (Figure 2.1a). This lesion can produce a number of signs and symptoms, including local pain, occipital headache and gross instability of the neck. Neurologic manifestations range from parasthesias to complete interference of neurologic function from the neck down. Gross instability of the neck can occur as a

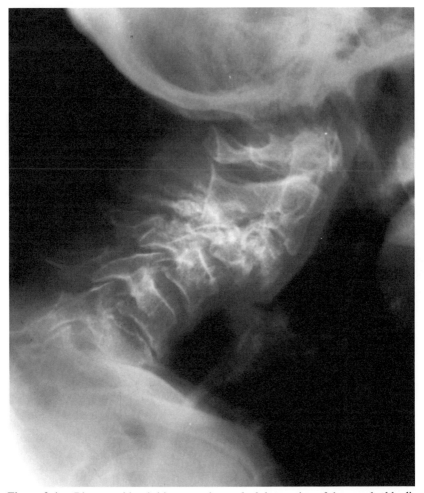

Figure 2.1a. Rheumatoid arthritis—note the marked destruction of the vertebral bodies.

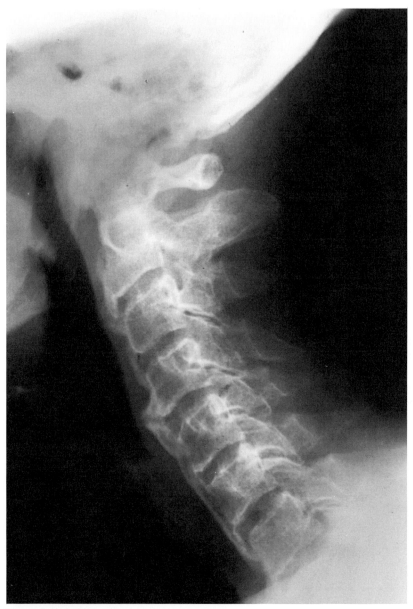

Figure 2.1b. Diffuse idiopathic spinal hyperostosis (DISH syndrome)—note the vertical appearance of the calcifications and osteophytes. There is a fracture of the upper portion of the hyperostotic segment.

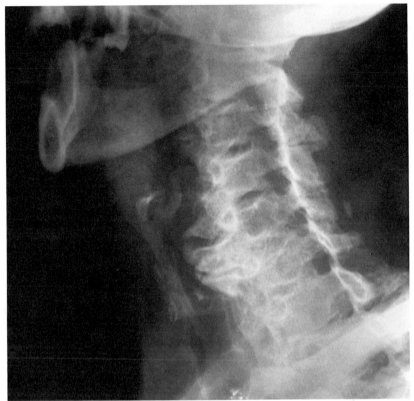

Figure 2.1c. Degenerative joint disease—note the horizontal extension of the osteophytes.

result of destruction of the ligaments and erosion of the odontoid process. Surgical stabilization is usually required in severe cases.

Pain in the shoulder can arise from local mechanical problems or may be referred from the neck. Many lesions that cause such pain are in the soft tissues. This topic will be discussed in more detail in a later chapter.

Primary muscle disease, such as polymyositis or dermatomyositis, described by a patient as pain in the muscles with any attempted motion is an uncommon condition. A more frequent disorder is fibromyalgia, which is characterized more by muscle aching than by pain.

In elderly patients, polymyalgia rheumatica is manifested as a marked muscle stiffness after a period of inactivity, such as in the morning following sleep. Patients must sometimes get out of bed by rocking themselves into the upright position. This condition is one of the few musculoskeletal disorders that can be diagnosed by a nonspecific laboratory test, a markedly elevated erythrocyte sedimentation rate.

Management of most soft-tissue and arthritic problems of the cervical spine is generally geared to relief of spasm of the paraspinal and spinal muscles. Useful medications include nonsteroidal anti-inflammatory drugs (NSAIDs) and muscle relaxants. The most useful muscle relaxant appears to be diazepam (2 mg one to three times daily) for a short course (three to five days). Drug abuse does not seem to occur with such short-term therapy. If a chronic occipital headache develops, phenytoin (100 mg three times daily) may be helpful.

In addition to medication, physical therapy, including hot packs, ultrasound and massage, is extremely beneficial in decreasing muscle spasm. Traction and soft cervical collars are usually not helpful and may cause further muscle atrophy and pain.

Transcutaneous nerve stimulation is beneficial in relieving pain and reducing the need for oral analgesics. Electrodes are placed at the appropriate trigger areas to interrupt the pain cycle.

DISORDERS OF THE LOWER BACK

Low-back pain is a prevalent health problem among inhabitants of industrialized countries of the West, where most studies of this problem have been conducted (4). Such studies indicate that up to 80 percent of the population will be affected at one time or another!

A well-planned study of low-back pain was carried out in Glostrup, Denmark; the study group consisted of people selected on the basis of various characteristics who were followed up for 12 months. The subjects were 60, 50, 40 or 30 years of age at the time of the initial examination. The participation rate of those selected was 82 percent; 449 men and 479 women comprised the group used for analysis. A questionnaire at 12 months was completed by 99 percent of the participants. A lifetime prevalence of about 62 percent was reported for the group, with a slight excess among the men. During the 12 months before the study began, about 45 percent of the participants reported having had such complaints; at the time of examination, 12 percent of the men and 15 percent of the women reported the complaints. The group with the maximal duration of symptoms (96 days) in the preceding period consisted of 60-year-old women; the lowest duration (20 days) was among 30-year-old men. As would be expected, heavy lifting was the most frequently reported cause of symptoms, and 60 percent of the participants (including housewives!) claimed that the lifting was related to their work. Women also ascribed the symptoms to menstruation. The only physical measurement that was significantly different in the group with symptoms was unequal leg length.

The question of hypermobility was brought up because of evidence that men with greater mobility in the lumbar spine may be at greater risk for the development of symptoms. A prior study has associated this factor only in women (6). However, in studies conducted by the author and his colleagues in Rochester to evaluate hypermobility, it was found that men had more hypermobility of the spine than did women.

The general conclusion of the author of this extensive Danish study of back pain was that "the more recently and frequently a person has had (low back pain) in earlier life, the more liable he or she will be to experience a new attack during the year to come."

It is clear that this syndrome will be the most frequent cause of back pain to bedevil primary-care physicians. Basic programs of care require a combination of therapies: bedrest, exercise, and therapy with an NSAID with or without a muscle relaxant agent.

Bedrest as initial therapy should be carried out for about one or two weeks. In elderly patients, strict bedrest should be limited to two to three days to help avoid the complications of prolonged bedrest, including deep-vein thrombosis, pneumonia, disuse atrophy, osteoporosis and incontinence. Patients should sleep on a firm but comfortable bed. A few patients obtain greater relief from the use of a support under the knees to keep them somewhat flexed. However, the author agrees with Quinet and Hadler (7) that prolonged, strict bedrest may not be advisable or adhered to by patients.

Analgesic agents, by controlling the pain, produce greater muscle relaxation. Although most muscle relaxants may help, the evidence for their effectiveness is not conclusive. The author believes that the dosage required for their maximal effect is such that side effects are frequent, necessitating discontinuation of therapy; however, this problem may be avoided by prescribing a short course of diazepam at a low dosage. Occasionally, adding a pure analgesic to an NSAID will afford greater relief. If there is muscle spasm, local application of heat may be effective. If heat fails to provide relief, application of cold is sometimes beneficial. Cold is an analgesic agent and can easily be applied, sometimes with less trouble than heat. For example, heat to the back can be provided by a heating pad, hot-water bottle, moist hot packs or a hot shower with the water drumming on the affected area. Unless heating pads are used with a timer or a shutoff device, they are dangerous to elderly patients. The author has seen an elderly patient who fell asleep with a heating pad, which burned the patient, leading to an untimely death. Moist heat is more penetrating than is dry heat, but it is more difficult to prepare and apply. The humble hot-water bottle has a safety feature in that it returns the temperature to an ambient level so that there is no danger of a patient falling asleep with a persistent local hotspot. Traction is not helpful in such cases.

In their excellent review on back pain, Quinet and Hadler have pointed out the self-limited nature of most cases of acute disease (7). They noted that 50 percent of patients feel better within one week, rising to about 80 percent in two weeks; about 90 percent feel better in about eight weeks. The author usually allows about 12 weeks for marked improvement to occur. The previously cited therapies can be used during this time frame with great benefit. Patients with

TABLE 2.1 Etiologic Bases of Back Pain

Ankylosing Spondylitis
Inflammatory Reiter's syndrome
  Reactive arthritis (chronic inflammatory bowel disease)
    Psoriatic arthritis
  Spondylosis
  Spondylolisthesis
  Diskitis
Osteomyelitis (acute, chronic, tuberculous, cocci)
  Degenerative apophyseal arthritis
  Congenital hypertrophic osteoarthropathy
Diffuse idiopathic skeletal hyperostosis
Prolapsed intervertebral disk
  Spinal stenosis
  Osteoporosis
  Osteomalacia
  Ochronosis
  Metabolic ochronosis
  Hyperparathyroidism
  Paget's disease
Traumatic fractures/dislocations
  Primary tumors
neoplastic/metastatic tumors
  Multiple myeloma

low-back pain lasting more than three months can be considered to have chronic disease.

If problems persist, a patient has chronic back disease, which can create subsequent problems. Patients may become depressed because the pain prevents them from functioning at work or even in activities of daily living. Table 2.1 lists the most common causes of back pain.

Inflammatory causes of back pain are those in which the primary disease is truly a spinal condition, such as ankylosing spondylitis. This disease starts in the sacroiliac joints. It may progress to involve the entire spine, causing ankylosis from the cervical spine to the sacrum. In the early stages, when there may be only minimal changes, the clinical signs and symptoms can be diagnostic. Ankylosing spondylitis is predominantly a disease of young men, starting in the teens and twenties, but has been encountered occasionally in men over age 50. The low-back pain can be relieved to some extent by exercise. Patients fall asleep without much difficulty and often wake up early in the morning. On awakening, they often obtain relief from their pain by lying on a hard surface (e.g., the floor) or sitting in a hard-backed chair. Such patients may also have pain that simulates sciatica. However, the pain may alternately affect either side, not showing the fixed pattern typically encountered with herniated intervertebral disks. Roentgenograms may demonstrate fuzziness in the sacroiliac joints, but this finding is not definitive. In elderly patients, however, it can be considered diagnostic. Roentgenograms may also demonstrate progression of the disease from the sacroiliac joints to involve the apophyseal joints, followed by the development of calcium deposits in the ligaments to produce the classical final appearance of "bamboo spine" (Figure 2.2). A number of subtle early changes are also visualized by roentgenography; examples are the erosion seen at the edges of the vertebral bodies and "squaring" of the vertebral bodies. Long treatises have been written on the roentgenographic changes seen in this disease, and it would be an educational experience for a physician to view such films in consultation with a radiologist to learn about these fine points.

Although more than 90 percent of patients with ankylosing spondylitis have human leukocyte antigen (HLA-B27), about 8 percent of the general population without the disease also carries this antigen. For this reason, antigen studies add little of clinical utility.

Management of ankylosing spondylitis is traditionally accomplished with an NSAID (excluding aspirin). Although therapy is usually effective in relieving pain and maintaining muscle function, it may affect the course of the disease. A retrospective study from Scandinavia indicates that persistent usage of an NSAID, even when a patient is apparently doing well without clinical manifestations, may inhibit progression of the disease (8).

Reiter's syndrome consists of the triad of nongonococcal urethritis, conjunctivitis and arthritis. However, it may also involve the nervous system, gastrointestinal tract and skin, creating major clinical manifestations. In mild cases, arthritis is combined with only one other component of the triad. Although generally considered a venereal condition, accompanied by a genital discharge, the syndrome can develop after a bout of bacterial dysentery. The latter form of reactive arthritis is most common in elderly patients. The offending organisms are *Shigella, Salmonella* and *Yersinia species.*

Involvement of the spine is usually restricted to the sacroiliac joints, creating low-back pain. The sacroilitis may be unilateral, in contrast to the bilaterality seen in ankylosing spondylitis. Other joints, particularly those of the legs, can be involved. In many cases, there are characteristic mucocutaneous lesions. Keratoderma blennorrhagicum is encountered most often, usually appearing on the feet, initially as small vesicles but later becoming confluent until there is a piling up of cornified skin. Such lesions are often indistinguishable from psoriasis. All these clinical features help pinpoint the cause of low-back pain in young male patients. However, the diagnosis can be difficult when the pain is due to an enteric pathogen in an elderly female patient. HLA-B27 antigen is carried by about 60 percent of such patients.

Like ankylosing spondylitis, Reiter's syndrome can occur intermittently. Bouts of genital discharge, severe keratoderma that makes walking difficult and low-back pain may be separated by periods of quiescence. Nonetheless, if the sacroiliac joints and lumbar spine demonstrate syndesmophytes, roentgenograms show persistence of this change during such periods. This form of the syndrome is the most common variant seen in the United States.

Management is the same as that used for ankylosing spondylitis; NSAIDs,

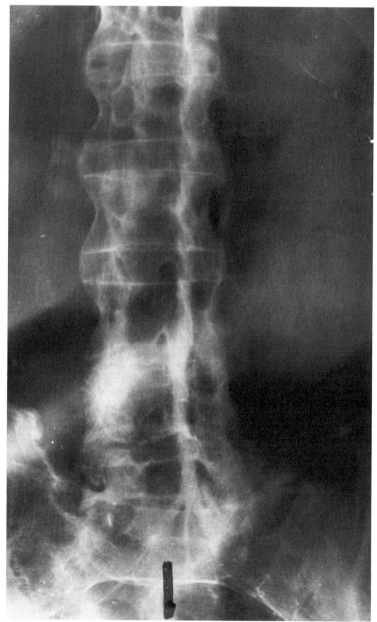

Figure 2.2. Ankylosing spondylitis showing the typical "bambooing" between vertebrae. Sacroiliac fusion is noted as well.

however, have not been reported to slow the progression of Reiter's syndrome. The author had a patient in whom urethritis, as manifested by a discharge, was the presenting clinical sign; the urethritis appeared to develop after intercourse. This observation lends credence to the claim that the disease is caused by *Chlamydia trachomatis* acquired in this manner, although this possibility has yet to be proved.

There are two major types of arthritis associated with chronic inflammatory bowel disease. Peripheral joint arthritis affects mostly the large joints and occurs in 10 to 20 percent of cases. About 7 percent of patients with ulcerative colitis or chronic regional ileitis (Crohn's disease) also have ankylosing spondylitis. Such patients carry the HLA-B27 antigen, and their ankylosing spondylitis probably is merely a coincident condition, although its development may be related to the arthritis. Whereas there are periods of remission and exacerbation corresponding to the relative severity of bowel complaints, the spondylitis has an independent clinical course. As for ankylosing spondylitis, the arthritis is managed with an NSAID.

The other major type is psoriatic arthritis accompanied by spondylitis. In this type, changes are observed in the spine more frequently than in the sacroiliac joints, according to Lambert and Wright (9).

These investigators found spondylitis in almost 50 percent of patients with peripheral arthritis. Ankylosing spondylitis occurs in about 5 percent of patients with psoriasis; such patients carry the HLA-B27 antigen and thus represent a subgroup in which there is overlap of the two diseases.

Another inflammatory cause of back pain is infection. The spine is particularly susceptible to acute bacterial infection because of the presence of a rich venous network known as Batson's plexus. Back pain of sudden onset after a urologic procedure should arouse suspicion of diskitis or osteomyelitis of the vertebral bodies. Chronic granulomatous infections, such as tuberculosis and coccidiomycosis, can also present with back pain. The delay from onset of the disease until a definitive diagnosis has been made can often be as long as 12 months.

Examination of a patient with infection in the back frequently demonstrates excruciating pain in the area of the involved vertebral bodies (most often the upper lumbar of midthoracic region), paravertebral spasm and hamstring spasm. Roentgenograms show irregularity of the subchondral bone plate of the adjacent vertebrae and, later, loss of the disk space and bony destruction (Figure 2.3). In cases of chronic infection, such as tuberculosis, severe destruction of a vertebral body can lead to an acute gibbous deformity and compression of the spinal cord (Figure 2.4). A paravertebral abscess may be demonstrated by computerized axial tomography.

Needle biopsy may be required for distinguishing infection from a malignant lesion or for obtaining tissue to allow definitive identification of the offending organism.

Management involves antibiotic therapy and immobilization of the spine in a body jacket. Clinical manifestations usually resolve within one or two weeks.

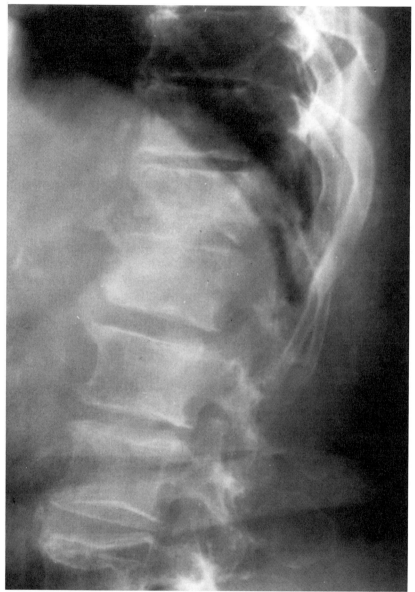

Figure 2.3. Osteomyelitis with discitis—beginning obliteration of the disc space with onset of destruction of the adjacent vertebrae.

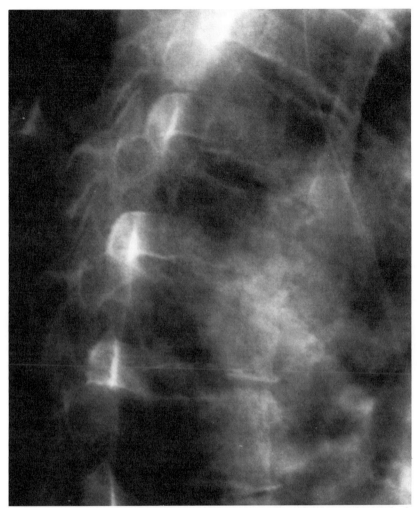

Figure 2.4. Tuberculosis of the spine—note the destruction of the thoracic vertebral body.

If there is a paravertebral abscess or acute neurologic deterioration, exploration of the area, drainage of the abscess, decompression and, in some cases, fusion are required.

Most of the degenerative and congenital conditions listed in Table 2.1 are usually encountered by orthopedic surgeons and not by rheumatologists. In almost all cases of low-back pain, the cause is diagnosed by the examining physician after roentgenograms have been obtained. This statement applies in particular to cases of spondylosis, spondylolisthesis and degenerative apophyseal arthritis and occasionally with prolapsed intervertebral disks (Figures 2.6–2.7).

In some patients with swollen ankles or wrists, careful examination reveals swelling and tenderness of the soft tissue proximal to the joint (not of the joint). The range of motion is normal or close to normal in most such cases. A consideration in the differential diagnosis here is hypertrophic osteoarthropathy. Again, the characteristic roentgenographic appearance of periostitis is a definitive finding. A similar clinical picture is encountered with sarcoidosis accompanied by periarthritis, which may be documented by a roentgenogram of the chest.

Diffuse idiopathic skeletal hyperostosis, also known as ankylosing hyperostosis or Forestier's disease, is often confused with classical ankylosing spondylitis. A major difference between these entities is the age at onset: Ankylosing spondylitis is mostly seen in young men, whereas ankylosing hyperostosis is a disease of the elderly. Again, roentgenograms are the definitive diagnostic study. The confusion between these entities is evident in reports that have described patients with the bamboo spine of ankylosing spondylitis but normal sacroiliac joints (10).

Yagan and Khan reviewed hundreds of cases of ankylosing spondylitis and did not find a single one with the classical changes in the spine and normal sacroiliac joints (10). Diffuse idiopathic skeletal hyperostosis is characterized by ossification of the anterior longitudinal ligament. There is also bony intervertebral bridging, a finding that can be distinguished from the syndesmophytes of ankylosing spondylitis.

Pain and disability are relatively minimal in ankylosing hyperostosis, unlike the situation in ankylosing spondylitis. However, therapy for the two conditions is similar, consisting of administration of an NSAID. In general, elderly patients (especially those over age 70) should initially be given half the recommended dosage. This approach can be effective and is safer in this age group. If relief of pain is inadequate after a few weeks, the dosage can be increased.

The most serious clinical sign of osteoporosis is fracture of the involved hip. Fractures of the spine occur chiefly in the thoracic and lumbar regions. Such compression fractures are due to the decreased mass of the vertebrae in these regions. The fractures may be asymptomatic, leading to kyphosis, or mild trauma or activity can produce a painful fracture. Back pain can usually be localized to the area of the fracture and may be so severe that it immobilizes the patient, who experiences difficulty finding a comfortable position. Any increase in intra-abdominal pressure, such as that associated with a bowel movement, creates pain. Bedrest usually affords relief but aggravates osteoporosis. The episodes sometimes resolve slowly but may recur.

Osteomalacia is not usually confined to the spine, sometimes resulting in myopathy and fractures of the long bones as well as diffuse bone pain.

Another disorder that can cause back pain is hyperparathyroidism, primary or secondary; in either case, there is the same degree of increased bone turnover. The roentgenographic demonstration of osteitis fibrosa cystica confirms the diagnosis. Other characteristic findings include hypercalcemia and hypophosphatemia.

Ochronosis is usually diagnosed on the basis of roentgenograms in patients with back pain and stiffness. This condition results from the deposition of the

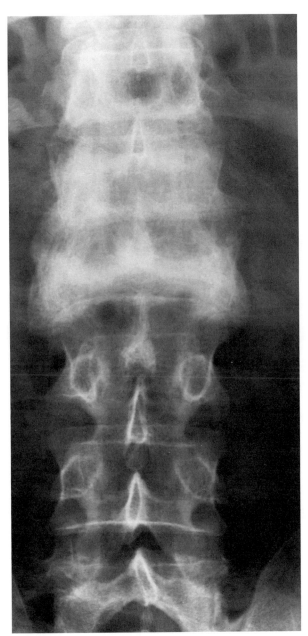

Figure 2.5. Paget's Disease of thoracic and lumbar spinal vertebrae.

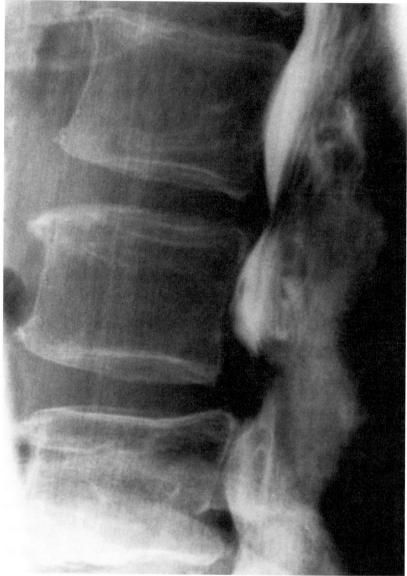

Figure 2.6. Intervertebral disc disease—the myelogram shows disc protrusion in two interspaces.

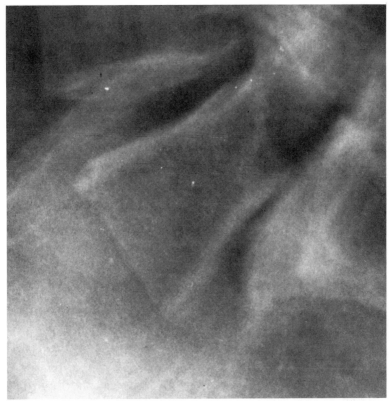

Figure 2.7. Spondylolisthesis of lumbar vertebrae—note the anterior displacement of the vertebral body.

pigment homogentisic acid in the articular cartilage, which is followed by the accumulation of calcium deposits in many intervertebral disks. In addition to turning black, the articular cartilage becomes brittle and shows osteoarthritic changes.

Although many patients with Paget's disease are asymptomatic, with the disease discovered as an incidental finding on roentgenograms, other patients present with severe pain. Thickening and coarsening of the trabecular pattern are pathognomonic roentgenographic findings (Figure 2.5).

In the author's experience in rheumatology clinic, the most helpful screening tests for elderly patients with back pain are the erythrocyte sedimentation rate and estimation of hemoglobin content. Patients with primary or metastatic tumors may show elevation of the sedimentation rate (30–40 mm/h) and the hemoglobin. Multiple myeloma usually induces a marked elevation of the sedimentation rate (to 80 to 100 mm per hour) and a prominent anemia (< 9 gm). Multiple myeloma also is accompanied by generalized osteoporosis and not by the localized lesions encountered with most primary and metastatic tumors.

This section has discussed the multifactorial basis of neck and back pain. It is evident that geriatricians must avoid the common error of defining a symptom as a disease. It is also important to recognize that the elderly are likely to have coexisting disorders. For example, virtually all elderly patients have some degree of spondylosis, but pain may be evidence of a new health problem, for example, myeloma, metastasis or infection. Neck and back pain thus are symptoms that should prompt a thorough investigation.

REFERENCES

1. Jayson, M.I.V. The inflammatory component of mechanical back problems. *Brit. J. Rheum.* 25:210–213, 1986.
2. Compere, E.L. The painful shoulder. *Amer. Med. Assoc.* 180:845–849, 1964.
3. Kankaanpaa, U., and Santavirta, S. Cervical spine involvement in rheumatoid arthritis. *Ann. Chir. Gynecol.* 74(Suppl. 198):117–121, 1985.
4. Kelsey, J.L., and White, A.A., III. Epidemiology and impact of low back pain. *Spine* 5:133–142, 1980.
5. Biering-Sorensen, F. A one-year prospective study of low back trouble in a general population. *Dan. Med. Bull.* 31:362–375, 1980.
6. Howes, R.G., and Isdale, I.C. The loose back: An unrecognized syndrome. *Rheumatol. Phys. Med.* 11:72–77, 1971.
7. Quinet, R.J., and Hadler, N.M. Diagnosis and treatment of backache. *Semin. Arthritis Rheum.* 8:261–287, 1979.
8. Boersma, J.W. Retardation of ossification of the lumbar vertebral column in ankylosing spondylitis by means of phenylbutazone. *Scand. J. Rheumatol.* 5:60–64, 1976.
9. Lambert, J.R., and Wright, V. Psoriatic spondylitis: A clinical and radiological description of the spine in psoriatic arthritis. *Q. J. Med.* 46:411–425, 1977.
10. Yagan, R., and Khan, M.A. Confusion of roentgenographic differential diagnosis between ankylosing hyperostosis (Forestier's disease) and ankylosing spondylitis. *Clin. Rheum.* 2:285–292, 1983.

Spinal Stenosis

Barry Kriegsfeld

A syndrome recognized with increasing frequency in elderly patients is associated with stenosis of the lumbar spine. The characteristic clinical features of this syndrome should alert physicians who care for such patients so that appropriate diagnostic studies can be carried out. This often misdiagnosed condition has distinctive anatomic, clinical and roentgenographic features. However, from the first recorded description of neurogenic claudication by Verbiest in 1949 (1) to the present era of magnetic resonance imaging, the diagnosis has eluded even the most experienced clinicians. Although neurogenic claudication and vascular claudication have a number of clinical similarities, which will be enumerated later, the two conditions have completely different pathophysiologic mechanisms.

An abnormality common to all elderly patients with neurogenic claudication is stenosis of the spinal canal. According to Pennal and Schatzker (2), there are only two etiologic bases of such stenosis: congenital narrowness of the canal in combination with further acquired narrowing and stenosis as a result of degenerative changes. The stenosis can be localized or multisegmental and involves appreciable narrowing of the anteroposterior diameter of the canal and extreme narrowing of the lateral recesses. The most frequently encountered constellation of changes in patients with this condition includes thickening of the laminae, enlargement of the ligamentum flavum, an absence of epidural fat, hypertrophy of the apophyseal joints, severe osteophytosis and a more horizontal orientation of the thickened laminae, allowing for marked indentation of the superior aspect of each lamina. The normally occurring lateral bony recess at the levels of L4 and L5, coupled with the more profound degenerative changes at these levels, predisposes L4 and L5 to be the sources of symptoms. Because of considerable variation in the anatomic structure of the lumbar spine, it is not unusual to find a well-defined lateral bony recess at L3 and even L2, so that stenosis at these levels is not uncommon. All these static abnormalities allow for predisposition to the syndrome of neurogenic claudication.

In addition to static anatomic abnormalities, one sees dynamic anatomic abnormalities that lead to a characteristic posture, namely, a stooped position for ambulation that becomes more pronounced as the condition progresses.

The author has thus termed this condition the "Groucho Marx syndrome." This posture can best be described as resulting from changes in the neural canal. Normally, the lumbar portion of the canal responds to extension by a buckling inward of the ligamentum flavum, an increase in the anterior length of the canal and a consequent decrease in its posterior length as well as a bulging of the posterior aspect of the disks into the canal, thus effectively decreasing the overall volume of the lumbar portion. On the other hand, flexion results in stretching of the ligamentum flavum, an increase in the posterior length of the canal and a consequent decrease in its anterior length as well as a decrease in the posterior aspect of the disks. The cross-sectional area of the nerve roots, which are being stretched, decreases, whereas the cross-sectional area of the nerve roots in the extended position (relaxed nerve roots) increases. These dynamic anatomic changes allow for the creation or alleviation of symptoms, as will be further explained (3).

The hallmark of neurogenic claudication associated with stenosis of the lumbar portion of the canal is pain, paresthesias or weakness associated with activity and alleviated to a greater or lesser degree by bending forward. Characteristically, patients are asymptomatic or relatively free of symptoms at rest or in the sitting position. With activity, such as walking, the symptoms arise after a variable period and are relieved by the previously mentioned maneuver. Not only is relief afforded by flexing, but more often than not, the relief is dramatic, produced simply by stopping walking and sitting or standing in a partially flexed position. The symptoms are therefore reminiscent of those of vascular claudication, but important differences exist that should lead the examiner to the proper diagnosis. Symptoms of unilateral neurogenic claudication should not lead the physician to exclude this diagnosis for Pennal and Schatzker found such symptoms in some of their patients.

The major clinical manifestations of pain, a motor deficit and a sensory deficit, the hallmarks of neurogenic claudication, can be differentiated from the findings associated with arterial insufficiency. A motor deficit in a patient with arterial insufficiency is a rare finding, but this problem may be interpreted as such by the patient in that a cramping tightness occurs after walking or exercise. A patient with neurogenic claudication may experience a motor deficit, but it is related to exercise and disappears with rest. A sensory deficit, although rarely or minimally associated with arterial insufficiency, is not an uncommon component of the constellation of symptoms of neurogenic claudication. The cramping pain associated with arterial insufficiency should be differentiated from the hyperpathic or dysesthetic pain associated with neurogenic claudication. Of course, pain in both instances is relieved by rest. The pain characteristically begins proximally and extends distally or begins distally and extends proximally in patients with neurogenic claudication. This so-called march of symptoms is distinctly absent in patients with arterial insufficiency. The pain in patients with neurogenic claudication is located in the back or in a sciatic distribution, whereas in those with arterial insufficiency, it is located in the muscles that are being exercised. Exercise pain, the hallmark of arterial insufficiency, may not be experienced by patients with neurogenic claudication.

Physical examination reveals important differences between the two conditions. Patients with arterial insufficiency usually have an arterial murmur, which is a rare finding in patients with neurogenic claudication. Moreover, the absence of or a decrease in the peripheral pulse should arouse suspicion of arterial insufficiency. The pulse of a patient with neurogenic claudication would most likely be normal. One must keep in mind that these two conditions affect patients in similar age groups, and their coexistence may cause diagnostic confusion. At rest, Lasègue's sign (straight leg raising) is normal in patients with neurologic involvement. One would expect that this sign would also be normal in patients with arterial insufficiency. The diagnostic confusion may be resolved if the examiner finds changes in the neurologic portion of the physical examination after exercise, which should suggest neurogenic claudication as the etiologic basis of the symptoms.

Pathophysiologic studies reveal a good correlation between sagittal narrowing of the spinal canal and symptoms of neurogenic claudication (4–6). Neurogenic claudication due to some other cause (neoplasia or marked protrusion of a disk) rarely is manifested by the distinctive symptom complex described previously (7).

In their classical study, Wilson and colleagues (8) described two distinct groups of patients in whom stenosis of the spinal canal resulted in different clinical syndromes. Although dynamic symptoms occur in all patients with intermittent neurogenic claudication, such symptoms develop in response to postural changes in one group. In the other group, symptoms arise only after exercise involving the legs. In the latter group, the symptoms appear to result from arterial insufficiency to the cauda equina, leading the author to term this condition "angina lumboris."

Symptoms of claudication that occur with changes in posture are clearly related to the neutral position, or lordosis, of the lumbar spine. Characteristically, patients bend forward to obtain relief of the symptoms, which takes place because this maneuver temporarily enlarges the spinal canal. Ehni (5) clearly demonstrated a marked change in the diameter of the lumbar portion of the canal during myelography. This observation leads the author to recommend that extension on the myelogram table be tried. It can make the examiner feel more secure in a diagnosis of postural claudication, especially if extension creates a total block.

Regarding ischemic claudication, the physician is faced with a differential diagnosis that includes neurogenic claudication and vascular claudication. As with vascular claudication, the appearance of neurologic symptoms in neurogenic cases is related to exercise much as angina pectoris is. The onset of symptoms is no doubt related to cauda equina ischemia. Experimental models have clearly shown the relationship of exercise to the rate of oxygen consumption in the cauda equina (9).

The radicular arteries that course from the lumbar arteries supply blood to the cauda equina. These end arteries have no appreciable collateral circulation, and therefore the syndrome rarely improves with time. Patients show marked functional impairment. The proper diagnosis and appropriate therapy often lead to gratifying results. Because the great ventral radicular artery of Adamkiewicz enters at the level of L1 or L2 or higher, the upper lumbar or thoracic spine is rarely involved. Therefore, the possibility that this syndrome might cause not only cauda equina ischemia but more extensive spinal cord ischemia remains slight.

Therapy is aimed at alleviating the claudication-like symptoms. Because most patients have symptoms of degenerative arthritis, they can experience severe back pain. Although decompression of the cauda equina affords some relief of back pain, it is more effective in relieving the leg symptoms. Before a patient consents to undergo a potentially limb-threatening and even life-threatening procedure, such as decompressive laminectomy, he or she should be informed of this fact. Many patients undergo decompressive laminectomy only to find that their morning backache and other symptoms of osteoarthritis persist.

In the author's experience, epidural corticosteroid blocks are rarely effective. Of course, the risk of undergoing a series of epidural corticosteroid blocks is small; for this reason, although the success rate is low, it seems a reasonable initial approach.

Decompressive lumbar laminectomy can be safely performed even in frail elderly patients and can lead to gratifying results. The procedure involves an extremely wide laminectomy and at least partial removal of the facet joints. The removal of ventral osteophytes seems an unnecessary procedure, in the author's opinion. During the operation, most surgeons note that the caudal sac migrates dorsally after the markedly thickened lamina and cauda equina are removed. Because of the long-standing compression in such patients, the dura is often thinned and adherent to overlying structures, making dissection difficult. Dural tears are common, necessitating meticulous repair. The author has found that repair with small sutures under magnification, followed by reinforcement with cyanoacrylate, affords the best chance of healing without persistent leakage of cerebrospinal fluid and the development of pseudomeningocele. The necessity of keeping the patient in a horizontal or head-down position for an extended period when a dural tear occurs makes surgical intervention even more dangerous and increases the risk for deep-vein thrombosis with pulmonary embolism. Prophylactic anticoagulation should be seriously considered in such patients.

An often confusing syndrome of neurologic origin has been discussed in a brief manner to alert physicians regarding its similarity to vascular claudication and to emphasize important features in the differential diagnosis. The observation of marked stenosis of the lumbar portion of the spinal canal in association with certain clinical findings can lead the clinician to a diagnosis of neurogenic claudication. Appropriate therapy can be instituted, after the lesion has been identified by one or more of the following procedures: computerized axial tomography of the lumbar spine with and without instillation of contrast medium, water-soluble myelography and, more recently, magnetic resonance imaging.

REFERENCES

1. Verbiest H. "Deonlwikkeling in de nuro chirurgische gednagingen." Amsterdam, Scheltema and Holkema, 1949, Vol. 28.
2. Pennal G.F. and Schatzker M. *Clinical Neurosurgery,* "Proceedings of the Congress of Neurological Surgeons," 1970. Baltimore, Williams & Wilkins, 1971, vol. 18, pp. 86–105.
3. Finneson, B.E. *Low Back Pain.* Stenosis of the Lumbar Spinal Canal, Philadelphia, Toronto, Lippincott, 1973.
4. Cooke, T.D.V., and Lehmann, P.O. Intermittent claudication of neurogenic origin. *Can. J. Surg.* 11:151–159, 1968.
5. Ehni, G. Spondylotic cauda equina radiculopathy. *Texas J. Med.* 61:746–752, 1965.
6. Verbiest, H. A radicular syndrome from developmental narrowing of the lumbar vertebral canal. *J. Bone Joint Surg. Brit. Vol.* 36-B:230–237, 1954.
7. Jennett, W.B. A study of 25 cases of compression of the cauda equina by prolapsed intervertebral discs. *J. Neurol. Neurosurg. Psychiatry* 19:109–116, 1956.
8. Wilson, C.B., Ehni, G., and Grollmus, Neurogenic intermittent claudication. *Clin. Neurosurg.* 18:62.
9. Larrabee, M.G. Oxygen consumption of excised sympathetic ganglia at rest and inactivity. *J. Neurochem.* 2:81–101, 1958.

Chapter 3

Franklin Kozin

Shoulder Pain

Pain and limitation of motion in the shoulder are among the most common problems that prompt patients to seek medical attention. In elderly patients, who often have other health problems, the impairment that results from shoulder problems may exceed that experienced by young patients to an appreciable extent. Prompt diagnosis and care are important in limiting disability.

The shoulder has evolved from a weight-bearing, supportive structure in lower animals to a highly mobile joint in human beings. This change has promoted hand (prehensile) function at the sacrifice of stability and explains the increased prevalence of shoulder disorders in man.

ANATOMY AND FUNCTION

The shoulder is composed of four joints that function in concert to produce movement in virtually all planes. These joints are the large glenohumeral joint and the acromioclavicular, sternoclavicular and scapulothoracic joints. The latter joint, although not a true synovial joint, is important in shoulder function.

The small sternoclavicular joint is formed by the first rib, clavicle and manubrium sterni. It contains a fibrocartilaginous intra-articular disk and is surrounded by a thick, fibrous capsule. The acromioclavicular joint also contains a small, often rudimentary, fibrocartilaginous intra-articular disk. These two joints allow the clavicle to rotate through its long axis, permitting elevation and depression of the shoulder girdle, as in shrugging the shoulder, or extension and flexion of the shoulder girdle, as in forward thrusting.

The glenohumeral joint is the major joint of the shoulder and is formed by the humerus and glenoid fossa of the scapula. The glenoid is shallow, although deepened to some extent by an encircling rim of cartilage, the labrum glenoidale. The surrounding articular capsule is loose and redundant. Stability of this joint is derived primarily from the surrounding short rotator muscles of the humerus. These muscles, which consist of the supraspinatus superiorly, the infraspinatus and teres minor posteriorly and the subscapular anteriorly, insert radially on

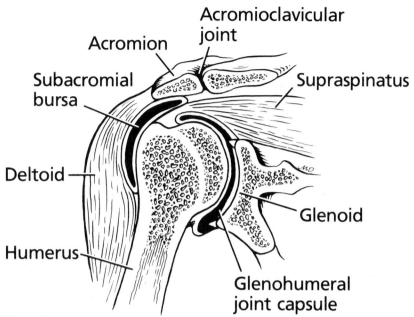

Figure 3.1. A cutaway view of the shoulder illustrates the relationship of the glenohumeral joint, subacromial bursa and rotator cuff (supraspinous tendon).

the head of the humerus through their conjoined tendons to form the rotator cuff (Figure 3.1).

The superior border of the rotator cuff is contiguous with the subacromial (subdeltoid) bursa. The large deltoid muscle overlies the bursa. Normally, the shoulder moves through a wide range of motion. It has been reported that motion may be reduced with increasing age; however, a recent study by Clarke did not support this observation (1).

EFFECTS OF AGING

Degenerative changes in the cartilage and other soft-tissue structures of the shoulder may be associated with aging, as was discussed in Chapter 1. DePalma reported that thinning and fibrillation were common in the glenoid cartilage but were less frequently observed in the humerus (2). Other investigators, however, have found little to no loss of integrity of the cartilage as a result of aging (3). Degenerative changes in the bicipital and rotator cuff tendons also have been reported to increase with age (4). Twenty-five percent of unselected subjects have attrition of the rotator cuff tendons by the fifth decade. The prevalence increases in subsequent decades (5).

Attritional changes in the soft tissues surrounding the glenohumeral joint probably explain the apparently increased incidence of tears of the rotator cuff tendons in the elderly population.

CLINICAL ASSESSMENT

The history and physical examination suggest the diagnosis in most patients with shoulder complaints. The initial evaluation is aimed at identifying the source and etiologic basis of the pain. Specifically, the examiner must determine first whether the pain is local or referred and then whether it is caused by a local, remote or systemic process.

The author has found it helpful to classify shoulder pain into two broad categories: intrinsic and extrinsic disorders (Table 3.1). Intrinsic conditions account for most causes of shoulder pain and reflect injury to the articular or musculotendinous structures surrounding the shoulder. Extrinsic pain may result from a systemic or generalized disorder, or it may be of viscerosomatic or neurovascular origin.

Intrinsic pain typically is localized to the deltoid muscle, glenohumeral joint or acromioclavicular joint. The most common source of intrinsic pain is disease in the rotator cuff, which is referred to the (sub)deltoid area. Patients usually relate their pain to shoulder movement and complain of interrupted sleep from pain induced by lying on the affected shoulder. Abnormalities in the physical examination usually confirm the diagnosis.

Extrinsic pain has a number of causes. Systemic or generalized arthritis is usually suggested by involvement of other joints and by constitutional symptoms (morning stiffness, fatigue, malaise, fever), signs of systemic disease and confirmatory laboratory studies. Myopathy and particularly polymyalgia rheumatica also should be suspected on the basis of associated systemic features.

Neurogenic pain is most commonly produced by radiculitis of a cervical nerve root due to formation of osteophytes or herniation of a disk. Pain in the shoulder may be caused by involvement of the C4, C5, C6 or C7 nerve roots.

TABLE 3.1 Intrinsic and Extrinsic Causes of Shoulder Pain

Intrinsic disorders
  Rotator cuff tendinitis/tear
  Bicipital tendinitis/tear
  Adhesive capsulitis
  Arthritis (local)
  Milwaukee shoulder syndrome
  Fibrositis/fibromyalgia
  Avascular necrosis
  Neoplasia
Extrinsic disorders
  Systemic or generalized arthritis
  Myopathy and polymyalgia rheumatica
  Metabolic and endocrine disorders
  Viscerosomatic pain (referred)
  Neurogenic pain
  Neurovascular pain
  Reflex sympathetic dystrophy

Although irritation of the C6 and C7 roots is encountered most often, involvement of one of these nerve root pairs is suggested by pain radiating into the forearm and thumb or middle finger, respectively. Less commonly, injury to the brachial plexus (blunt or penetrating trauma, traction injury, inflammation) or peripheral nerves may be manifested by shoulder pain.

Viscerosomatic pain is usually referred from an intrathoracic or intra-abdominal source. It is important to recognize such sources of pain so as not to miss a potentially serious medical or surgical condition. Pain from diaphragmatic irritation (pulmonary infection or infarction, subdiaphragmatic abscess) may result in pain referred to the trapezius ridge. Pain from disease in the liver or gallbladder may be referred to the (right) scapular area. The pain of myocardial infarction or ischemia is usually referred to the (left) pectoral area and ulnar aspect of the arm.

The pain of neurovascular and reflex sympathetic dystrophy (shoulder-hand syndrome) also may be most prominent in the shoulder and arm.

The physical examination confirms the diagnosis and helps pinpoint the source of pain. The shoulder should be examined with the patient sitting or standing and unclothed to the waist to permit thorough inspection and comparison of anatomic and functional symmetry. It is often useful to watch the patient remove his or her shirt or blouse in assessing shoulder function. The patient's habitus and posture also should be noted. The shoulders should be inspected for asymmetry, bony or soft-tissue swelling and deformity. Palpation may reveal specific areas of tenderness, suggesting arthritis in the glenohumeral, acromioclavicular or sternoclavicular joint, inflammation of the bicipital or rotator cuff tendons or fibrositis.

After these observations have been made, the range of shoulder motion should be evaluated (Figure 3.2). The patient is asked to begin with the arms relaxed and at the sides. He or she is then asked to elevate the arms forward over the head (flexion) and directly backward (extension) and to elevate the arms outward, over the head (abduction) and across the body (adduction). The patient is then asked to abduct the arms to a 90 degree angle, bend the elbows and move the hands upward (external rotation) and downward (internal rotation). Pain during these maneuvers (a painful arc) may indicate tendinitis. Resistance to the performance of these maneuvers on the part of the examiner also may help isolate the specific musculotendinous groups involved. Assessment of the passive range of motion may be especially helpful in patients with limitation of active motion.

RADIOGRAPHIC INVESTIGATION

Standard plain radiographs usually consist of anteroposterior views in internal and external rotation. Additional views may be obtained when indicated by the clinical history or when required for visualization of the scapula or acromioclavicular or sternoclavicular joint. Arthritis in the shoulder girdle joints, fracture,

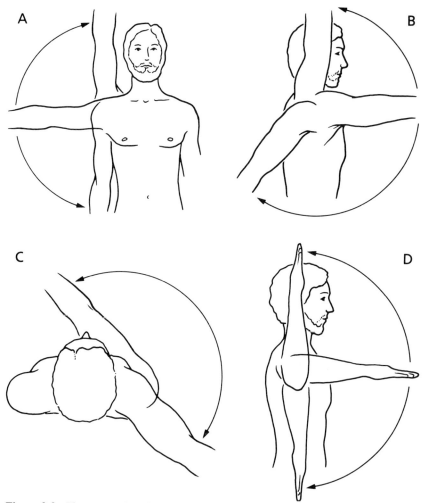

Figure 3.2. The range of motion of the normal shoulder is shown and is part of the physical examination of the shoulder. A, abduction and adduction; B, flexion and extension; C, horizontal flexion and horizontal extension; D, internal and external rotation.

dislocation and calcium deposits in the soft tissue may be seen. Osteitis with sclerosis, periostitis and cyst formation in the greater tuberosity are often encountered in patients with degenerative tendinitis.

Shoulder arthrography is particularly helpful in diagnosing tears in the rotator cuff tendons, abnormalities of the bicipital tendons and adhesive capsulitis (Figure 3.1). These changes will be more completely discussed in the sections that follow. Recent studies have suggested that sonography and magnetic resonance imaging may be useful in identifying rotator cuff lesions.

PAINFUL SHOULDER CONDITIONS

Intrinsic Disorders

ROTATOR CUFF LESIONS

Degenerative changes in the rotator cuff tendons frequently occur in the "aging" shoulder, as has been noted. Clinical features depend on the acuteness and severity of the problem.

The typical patient with rotator cuff tendinitis is a man in the fifth decade or older who works as a laborer and localizes his complaints to the dominant arm. However, women and men with sedentary lifestyles are not spared, especially with the increasing interest in fitness and exercise in our society.

Such patients describe a dull, aching pain in the shoulder that is difficult to localize; many patients point to the deltoid area. The pain may radiate down the arm as far as the hand, but this pattern is uncommon in the author's experience. Patients report that the pain is worse at night.

Physical examination may disclose tenderness of the affected tendon(s). Because supraspinous tendinitis is encountered most frequently, there is tenderness at or just proximal to the insertion of this tendon at the greater tuberosity. A painful arc is usually noted with abduction between angles of 60 and 120 degrees. Less commonly, and with involvement of other rotator cuff tendons, pain may occur with other movements of the shoulder. By resisting active motion on the part of the patient, additional information may be obtained. This approach is particularly helpful for isolating early or mild supraspinous tendinitis and differentiating it from arthritis in the glenohumeral or acromioclavicular joint. The patient is asked to abduct the arm to a 90 degree angle and hold it against downward pressure. Pain in the subdeltoid area suggests supraspinous tendinitis. Impingement syndrome, in which the supraspinous tendon is pinched between the head of the humerus and the acromion, may be recognized by this method, especially when pain is induced by resisted motion in 90 degrees of abduction and 45 to 60 degrees of horizontal flexion. The passive range of motion is normal, and muscle strength is minimally or not reduced.

Radiographic studies may demonstrate degenerative changes in the area surrounding the greater tuberosity with cyst formation, sclerosis and periosteal reaction.

Management of degenerative rotator cuff tendinitis is directed at relief of pain, improvement and maintenance of function, early rehabilitation, avoidance of complications (adhesive capsulitis or reflex sympathetic dystrophy) and prevention of recurrent pain. The basic conservative approach is outlined in Table 3.2.

For patients with an acutely painful shoulder, rest is essential. Immobilizing the arm in a sling with the shoulder in partial adduction is sometimes helpful. A patient should be encouraged to exercise once or twice daily; initially, exercise should consist only of "pendulum swings," in which the patient rocks the

TABLE 3.2   Conservative Regimen for Management of Shoulder Pain

1. Rest
    a. Severe pain with limited motion: complete rest
    b. Moderate pain: modified rest/mild exercise
    c. Mild pain: active exercise
2. Physical therapy
    a. Ice helpful in most patients; heat, or alternatively ice and heat, occasionally necessary
    b. Sonography with or without topical use of a corticosteroid
3. Medications
    a. Nonsteroidal anti-inflammatory drug
    b. Analgesic agent
4. Local injection of a corticosteroid

body while allowing the hanging arm to swing back and forth gently. In cases of a less painful shoulder, a patient is instructed to keep the arm below shoulder level, and daily range-of-motion exercises are prescribed to maintain and increase shoulder mobility. Although rest is important, early mobilization is essential to prevent such complications as adhesive capsulitis and reflex sympathetic dystrophy.

Physical therapy may provide considerable assistance to a patient in monitoring his or her exercise program and in using ice and heat modalities. Ultrasound may be beneficial, and topical corticosteroids administered under guidance with ultrasound may provide mild control of inflammation locally.

Analgesic and anti-inflammatory medications are used to control the pain. The author prescribes a salicylate or a nonsteroidal anti-inflammatory drug (NSAID) and supplements this agent with a simple or narcotic analgesic medication as needed.

If these measures fail to control the pain within two to four weeks, it is appropriate to consider local injection of a corticosteroid. The author has found it helpful to inject 2 to 3 ml of 1% lidocaine in the subacromial space or at the site of greatest tenderness and reassess the physical findings. This approach helps localize the best area for injection of the corticosteroid and illustrates the expected benefits to the patient. The shoulder is then injected with 20 to 40 mg of prednisolone tertiary butyl acetate, 20 to 80 mg of methylprednisolone acetate or an equivalent preparation admixed with 1 to 2 ml of 0.25 to 0.5 percent bupivacaine. Use of a local corticosteroid is not without potentially serious adverse reactions, such as the effects of systemic absorption, the risk for infection and the tendency to reduce tensile strength in the tendon, leading to the possibility of rupture.

Persistence of shoulder pain after four to six weeks of conservative therapy is uncommon in cases of tendinitis and should prompt a thorough reevaluation. Arthrography should be considered to rule out the possibility of a rotator cuff tear.

CALCIFIC TENDINITIS

Calcific tendinitis occurs equally in both sexes and in the dominant and nondominant shoulders, and it often affects persons with sedentary lifestyles. These observations suggest that the etiologic basis of calcific tendinitis differs from that of degenerative tendinitis. As in degenerative tendinitis, the supraspinous tendon is most commonly affected in patients with calcific tendinitis; however, more than one affected site and bilateral involvement are not uncommon occurrences.

The clinical manifestations of this condition may be indistinguishable from those of degenerative tendinitis, especially when the calcium deposits are localized. The deposits occasionally rupture into the subacromial bursa, producing an acutely painful shoulder, which the patient holds rigidly in a neutral position (Figure 3.2). It may prove impossible to examine the shoulder effectively.

Radiographs may reveal calcium deposits in the affected tendon or in the subacromial bursa (Figure 3.3).

Therapy for this condition is identical to that used for degenerative tendinitis unless the calcium deposits have ruptured into the bursa. The latter event should be dealt with as an acute crystal-induced process and may necessitate systemic administration of a corticosteroid. It is occasionally useful to attempt to mobilize or remove the calcium deposits, especially in patients with persistent or recurrent problems. The calcium may be removed by needling the affected area in an effort to aspirate the material; however, the needling process may induce a

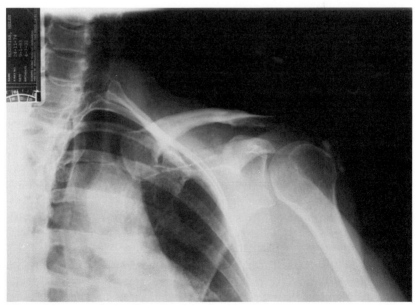

Figure 3.3. A standard radiograph of the shoulder demonstrates calcific tendinitis.

local reaction that promotes removal of the calcium. Surgical removal of calcium may be necessary in patients with recalcitrant deposits.

ROTATOR CUFF RUPTURE

Rotator cuff tears are not rare occurrences, particularly in elderly patients. In young patients, considerable force is needed to tear the rotator cuff tendons; most cases are the result of direct trauma, falls or athletic stress. In elderly patients, tears are idiopathic or occur in response to minor trauma. Tears may be partial or complete, in which case they involve the full thickness of the cuff. Partial tears usually affect the undersurface of the cuff, causing fraying, or partial-thickness tears.

The classical history of a fall accompanied by sudden pain and limitation of shoulder motion readily suggests the diagnosis. Persistence of shoulder pain in an elderly patient initially thought to have degenerative tendinitis often leads to further evaluation and diagnosis. The examination may reveal several findings that should lead the clinician to suspect a tear. Atrophy of the supraspinous fossa and weakness of the shoulder extensor muscles are often encountered. A useful maneuver is to instruct the patient to abduct the arm passively to a 90 degree angle and release it; patients with complete rotator cuff tears are unable to maintain the position and the arm drops to the side, the "drop arm sign."

A plain radiograph may be normal or may show changes that resemble those seen in degenerative tendinitis. Narrowing of the subacromial space is a useful radiographic sign of attrition in the rotator cuff or of a chronic tear. Complete tears are confirmed by arthrography; contrast medium is injected into the glenohumeral joint and is observed to extrude into the subacromial bursa (Figure 3.4). Partial tears may be visualized with double-contrast arthrography. Recent data suggest that sonography and magnetic resonance imaging may identify rotator cuff tears.

Therapy should be instituted as soon as possible to repair or limit the extent of the tear. Early surgical repair is advisable in cases of acute, complete tears. In cases of chronic tears, conservative management may be adequate for controlling symptoms with minimal impairment of function. Injection of a corticosteroid should be avoided as such drugs may weaken the remaining tendon structure and predispose to a recurrence. Surgical repair may be necessary, even in patients with chronic tears, but complete relief of pain and recovery of function should not be expected. Recently, arthroscopic debridement of the shoulder has been utilized to provide symptomatic relief with a much shorter rehabilitation period.

BICIPITAL TENDINITIS

There may be involvement of the bicipital tendon within the joint or in the bicipital groove beyond the point where the tendon exits the joint capsule. Although tendinitis is the most common problem, rupture or dislocation also occurs.

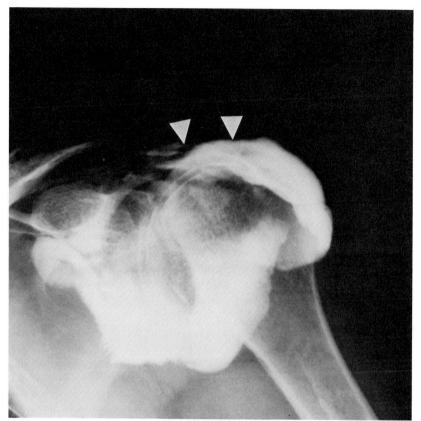

Figure 3.4. An arthrogram of the shoulder reveals constrast medium within the subacromial bursa (arrows), indicating a complete rotator cuff tear.

Bicipital tendinitis produces pain in the anterior aspect of the shoulder, and the pain may radiate down the arm and into the proximal portion of the forearm. Examination typically discloses tenderness of the bicipital tendon. Provocative maneuvers help confirm the diagnosis. Pain along the course of the tendon is produced by resisted supination of the forearm (Yergason's sign) or by resisted flexion. Rupture of the tendon leads to a (''Popeye'') bulge in the biceps muscle and absence of a palpable tendon. Radiographs are usually normal.

Therapy is similar to the regimen outlined in Table 3.2. Surgical intervention is rarely indicated, even in patients with ruptures.

ADHESIVE CAPSULITIS
This condition also known as frozen shoulder or shoulder periarthritis, is a unique disorder. It may develop spontaneously, or it may complicate shoulder

pain of some other etiologic basis. Adhesive capsulitis is characterized by poorly localized pain in the shoulder and loss of mobility. It is more common in women than in men, tends to occur in the fifth and later decades and is more frequently encountered in patients with diabetes mellitus than in those without this disorder. Physical examination shows diffuse tenderness around the shoulder. There is marked limitation of all shoulder motion (as opposed to tendinitis, which usually affects only elevation). Local infiltration of an anesthetic fails to improve the range of motion and further distinguishes this condition from tendinitis.

Plain radiographs demonstrate only localized osteopenia after at least four to six weeks of symptoms. Arthrography may reveal a reduction of joint volume.

Therapy is most effective when initiated early. A conservative approach is warranted for the first two to three weeks and should include active range-of-motion exercises and use of an NSAID and an analgesic. Local or systemic injection of a corticosteroid may be effective if the conservative regimen is unsuccessful (6). The physician may give a local injection consisting of 25 ml of sterile normal saline, 3 ml of 1 percent lidocaine and 20 to 80 mg of prednisone or methylprednisone or administer a drug systemically, as described for reflex sympathetic dystrophy (6).

ARTHRITIS
Arthritis in the shoulder is uncommon as an isolated process, although virtually any form of generalized arthritis or systemic rheumatic disease may affect the joints in this area. Osteoarthritis or degenerative arthritis may be encountered in the acromioclavicular joint or, less commonly, in the sternoclavicular or glenohumeral joint. Septic arthritis may develop insidiously, especially in elderly or debilitated patients.

MILWAUKEE SHOULDER SYNDROME
This syndrome is a distinctive condition originally recognized in the shoulders (7) but more recently identified in the knees and other joints. It is seen primarily in elderly patients, who describe moderate to severe pain in the shoulder associated with loss of motion. Physical examination often reveals a large synovial effusion and joint tenderness. There is marked limitation of motion (60 degrees or less) with flexion, abduction and rotation. Instability is occasionally noted in the glenohumeral joint. This syndrome appears identical to that described by Neer and colleagues, who termed it "cuff tear arthropathy" (8).

Radiographs invariably demonstrate advanced degenerative changes (Figure 3.5). Upward migration of the head of the humerus into or subjacent to the acromion is often seen. Soft-tissue calcium deposits are observed in about 40 percent of patients. Large rotator cuff tears have been reported in all patients. Formation of osteophytes is not a prominent change despite marked narrowing of the joint space and bony changes in the head of the humerus, suggesting that this syndrome may not be an osteoarthritic condition.

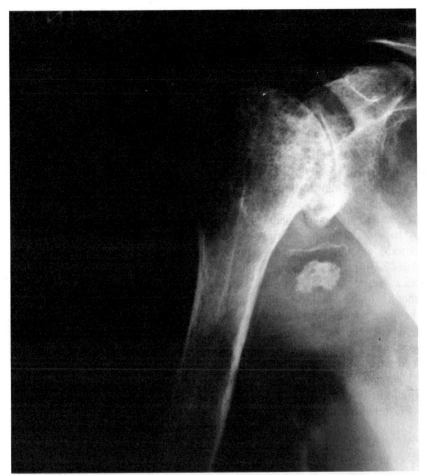

Figure 3.5. A radiograph from a patient with Milwaukee shoulder syndrome shows narrowing of the glenohumeral joint space, sclerosis and mild cystic degeneration of the head of the humerus. There also is a loose body within the joint inferiorly.

Analysis of synovial fluid usually reveals mild leukocytosis (fewer than 1000 leukocytes per cubic millimeter of blood). Hydroxyapatite (basic calcium phosphate) crystals are almost invariably seen and appear to have an important role in the pathogenesis of this syndrome (9).

Threapy is difficult and often unsatisfactory. The conservative approach discussed previously may be helpful. Surgical intervention has been advocated by Neer and colleagues, who have obtained encouraging preliminary results (8).

FIBROSITIS (fibromyalgia, myofascial syndrome)
This common rheumatic condition may develop at any age. Most patients are women. It is characterized by aching pain in the upper back, shoulder girdle,

neck and trapezius musculature, although most patients describe shoulder pain. The pain is often worse in the morning and may be associated with stiffness lasting several hours. Physical or emotional stress may exacerbate the pain. In severe cases, patients describe deep burning pain in the back, chest or upper arms and may report numbness or tingling in these areas. Sleep may be described as fitful or frankly interrupted two or more times during the night. Patients feel fatigued on arising.

Tenderness is characteristically noted in the upper back, neck, chest, buttocks, lateral epicondyles and knees. The physical examination is often otherwise normal. However, fibrositis may develop secondary to persistent pain syndromes, such as cervical spondylosis, rheumatoid arthritis and shoulder tendinitis.

Management may be difficult, especially in patients how have had long-standing pain. In many instances, the pain has been ignored by the patient or misdiagnosed by a physician unfamiliar with this condition, and the patient may be accused of malingering. Reassurance and thorough discussion of the syndrome are important; it is helpful to provide written material (magazine articles, Arthritis Foundation publications) to "prove" that the pain derives from a "real" problem. Various treatment regimens have been advocated. The author has found that the combination of an NSAID and a tricyclic antidepressant at bedtime is effective in many patients. The latter drug should be given at a low dosage and used with caution, especially in elderly patients; a thorough understanding of the side effects of such drugs is essential for their safe and effective use. Physiotherapy in which application of heat or cold, gentle massage, exercise and a reconditioning program are prescribed progressively may be helpful. In certain patients, biofeedback or transcutaneous nerve stimulation may be effective alone or in combination with the aforementioned approaches.

AVASCULAR NECROSIS

Avascular necrosis of the shoulder is an uncommon condition, especially as an isolated problem. It may occur in patients with involvement of other joints and usually is encountered as a complication of connective-tissue disorders, corticosteroid therapy or alcoholism.

NEOPLASIA

Primary and secondary neoplastic disorders may affect the shoulders. Although such disorders are infrequently the cause of unexplained shoulder pain, they should be kept in mind during evaluation. Radiography or bone scanning usually assists in the diagnosis.

Extrinsic Shoulder Disorders

GENERALIZED OR SYSTEMIC ARTHRITIS

Generalized or systemic arthritis may involve the shoulder joints, as discussed elsewhere in this chapter. In such instances, the diagnosis of shoulder pain is usually straightforward. However, sudden or disproportionate pain in a shoulder should prompt further investigation because an intrinsic disorder may be complicating an underlying problem. Indeed, an inflamed or "arthritic" shoulder may be more susceptible to partial or complete tears of the rotator cuff, tendinitis or septic arthritis. The latter condition may develop insidiously in patients with rheumatoid arthritis, subacute bacterial endocarditis or septicemia and in those treated with corticosteroids. Elderly patients appear to be especially susceptible to this problem.

MYOPATHY AND POLYMYALGIA RHEUMATICA

A complaint of shoulder weakness or pain should prompt the physician to consider these conditions. Polymyalgia rheumatica is a disease of the elderly, occurring mostly after age 55. It is more frequently encountered in women than in men and predominates in white patients. Pain in the shoulders, neck, upper arms, back and thighs may be severe and usually is of sudden onset, although it may develop insidiously. Morning stiffness is marked in the proximal portion of the shoulders and hip girdles but usually spares the more-distal joints, in contrast to rheumatoid arthritis. Constitutional symptoms, including generalized malaise, anorexia, lethargy, weight loss and fevers are not uncommon occurrences.

Physical examination may be unremarkable or may reveal mild inflammatory arthritis, limitation of shoulder or hip motion or abnormalities in the temporal or peripheral arteries (in patients with associated giant-cell arteritis).

Laboratory tests usually demonstrate mild to moderate anemia and a prolonged erythrocyte sedimentation rate.

In view of the nonspecific clinical and laboratory findings, careful evaluation is essential. The differential diagnosis includes rheumatoid arthritis, multiple myeloma, fibrositis and occult cancer.

Management should be initiated with 10 to 30 mg of prednisone (or its equivalent) daily (5 mg three or four times daily is a reasonable starting dosage). A dramatic response should be expected within three to seven days; if such a response is not observed, the diagnosis must be reassessed. After several weeks, the dosage should be tapered to a maintenance level of 5 to 10 mg in the morning and adjusted according to the erythrocyte sedimentation rate and symptoms.

VISCEROSOMATIC PAIN

Pain referred to a shoulder from a pathologic process in the thorax or abdomen is not a rare occurrence. Sites of referred pain are discussed in the preceding sections.

NEUROGENIC PAIN

Neurogenic pain is usually due to cervical radiculopathy (see Chapter 2) or brachial plexopathy. Metastatic cancer, Pancoast's tumors and lymphoproliferative disorders may directly involve the brachial plexus, causing shoulder pain. Management of the underlying condition is necessary.

NEUROVASCULAR PAIN AND REFLEX DYSTROPHY

These conditions are relatively uncommon. The neurovascular pain that accompanies thoracic outlet syndrome is characterized by a deep aching in a shoulder or an arm, especially when the arm is being used above the level of the head. Physical examination may demonstrate reduced radial artery pulses with provocative (thoracic outlet) maneuvers (6).

Reflex sympathetic dystrophy is a serious condition that may develop after trauma to an arm; alternatively, it may be a complication of hemiparesis, myocardial infarction, cervical spondylosis and other conditions often seen in elderly patients.

This nervous system disturbance may be associated with shoulder pain in patients with a variant of shoulder-hand syndrome. Patients describe severe pain, usually a burning sensation, especially in a hand or foot. The pain may be accompanied by swelling, tenderness and vasomotor changes (10); dystrophic skin changes also may be seen. Radiographs often assist in the diagnosis, demonstrating patchy osteopenia in the affected limb. Bone scans may reveal increased radionuclide uptake in periarticular tissues of the involved limb (11).

Early therapy is essential for controlling reflex sympathetic dystrophy. The most effective therapy is systemic injection of a corticosteroid (6,10) or chemical or surgical sympathetic nerve blockade (6).

REFERENCES

1. Clarke, G.R. Measurement in shoulder problems. *Rheumatol. Rehabil.* 15:191–193, 1976.
2. DePalma, A.F. *Surgery of the Shoulder,* ed. 2. Philadelphia, Lippincott, 1973, pp. 100–137.
3. Meachim, G. Effect of age on the thickness of adult articular cartilage at the shoulder joint. *Ann. Rheum. Dis.* 30:43–46, 1971.
4. Brewer, B.J. Aging of the rotator cuff. *Amer. J. Sports Med.* 7:102–110, 1979.
5. Moseley, H.F. *Shoulder Lesions,* ed. 3. Edinburgh, Churchill Livingstone, 1960.
6. Kozin, F. Painful shoulder and reflex sympathetic dystrophy syndrome, in McCarty, D.J., Jr. (ed.): *Arthritis and Allied Conditions,* ed. 10. Philadelphia, Lea & Febiger, 1985, pp. 1091–1120.
7. McCarty, D.J. Milwaukee shoulder: Association of microspheroids containing hydroxyapatite crystals, active collagenase and neutral protease with rotator cuff defects. I. Clinical aspects. *Arthritis Rheum.* 24:464–473, 1981.
8. Neer, C.S., Craig, E.V., and Fukuda, H. Cuff tear arthropathy. *J. Bone Joint Surg.* 69A:1232–1244, 1983.
9. Halverson, P.B. Milwaukee shoulder: Association of microspheroids containing hydroxyapatite crystals, active collagenase and neutral protease with rotator cuff defects. II. Synovial fluid studies. *Arthritis Rheum.* 24:474–483, 1981.

10. Kozin, F., McCarty, D.J., Sims, J., and Genaut, H.K. The reflex sympathetic dystrophy syndrome. I. Clinical and histologic studies: Evidence for bilaterality, response to corticosteroids, and articular involvement. *Amer. J. Med.* 60:321–331, 1976.
11. Kozin, F., Genant, H.K., Bekerman, C., and McCarty, D.J. The reflex sympathetic dystrophy syndrome. II. Roentgenographic and scintigraphic evidence of bilaterality and periarticular accentuation. *Amer. J. Med.* 60:332–338, 1976.

Chapter 4

Robert L. Wilson
David Haueisen

Hand and Wrist

Management of hand and wrist problems in elderly patients may be a formidable challenge for family practitioners, internists and orthopedists. Disease of or injury to the distal portion of an arm might create temporary difficulty for a young patient but is more likely to represent a serious situation for an elderly patient. Sudden inability to use a hand renders many elderly patients incapable of the activities of daily living. The goal of the physician in such instances is prompt diagnosis and treatment to allow elderly patients to regain at least partial use of the affected hand and, if possible, normal arm function.

More often, physicians are called on to manage chronic degenerative conditions that have gradually decreased the ability to function. A patient's specific needs and the functional loss must be carefully considered before any treatment is undertaken. Even when drug therapy or surgical intervention is not indicated, physicians can offer elderly patients useful assistance. Programs that teach patients how to protect joints are available, as are a number of inexpensive self-help aids and tools that assist with buttoning clothes, eating and grooming needs (1).

The care of elderly patients with hand problems involves special considerations. Not only do affected joints tend to become stiff, but also adjacent joints (2). A treatment regimen that leads to healing of a fracture but at the cost of decreased mobility in the adjacent joints must be considered a failure (3).

Management of a given hand problem is identical in elderly and young patients. Hand fractures take the same time to heal in any patient regardless of age (4,5). The basic principles in the management of hand fractures are accurate reduction, active motion of the uninvolved fingers, elevation of the hand to prevent edema and early protected motion when the fracture becomes consolidated. Space does not permit a detailed discussion of the management of specific fractures or small-joint injuries.

COLLES' FRACTURE

The most common fracture in patients over age 50 involves the distal portion of the radius and is named after Abraham Colles. The distal fragment is displaced dorsally, often in association with shortening and angulation of the radius (Figure 4.1A).

The injury is caused by a fall on an outstretched hand with the wrist extended. The fracture begins on the palmar surface of the radius and propagates dorsally, often compacting the dorsal portion to produce comminution. Colles' fractures are typically managed by closed reduction, which is achieved after anesthesia by traction and disimpaction of the fracture, followed by volar displacement of the distal fragment. Reduction can be maintained by means of a plaster splint or cast applied with the wrist held slightly flexed and in ulnar deviation. Extreme flexion and pronation of the wrist are contraindicated because these movements may lead to compression of the median nerve and stiffness of the fingers (6).

Maintaining precise reduction is difficult because collapse or settling occurs as part of the normal healing process in all Colles' fractures. When dorsal-radial comminution takes place (a more frequent occurrence in elderly than in young patients), the fracture may revert to its original, displaced position after the initial reduction. Unstable fractures and ones that redisplace can be managed by a distraction technique (7). One such method places pins through the second and third metacarpal bones distally and through the ulna proximally. Thereafter, the pins are incorporated into a plaster cast to maintain the corrected position of the fracture. A newer technique is the use of an external fixation device (8,9). Both methods allow unrestricted motion of the elbow and fingers. Colles' fractures are usually sufficiently healed by six to eight weeks to allow removal of the cast or fixation apparatus (Figure 4.1B).

Complications of Colles' fractures occur in about 30 percent of cases and deserve considerable attention (10,11). Age and mechanism of injury bear no relationship to the incidence of such complications. Problems that develop after Colles' fractures can be classified as early or late (Table 4.1). Complications are directly related to the precision of fracture reduction (12). Thus, every reasonable attempt should be made to achieve anatomic alignment of the fracture fragments. However, overzealous attempts to maintain a near-perfect reduction are not justified in elderly patients.

The most devastating problem that can occur after a Colles' fracture is stiffness within the small joints of the hand. Stiffness can result from edema, or it may develop if a plaster cast extends too far distally, blocking full motion of the fingers or prohibiting the patient from exercising appropriately. Motion of the fingers, elbow and shoulder must be carefully monitored throughout the treatment period (13). If a patient begins to lose motion, an exercise program directed by an experienced hand therapist may be able to reverse this change (14).

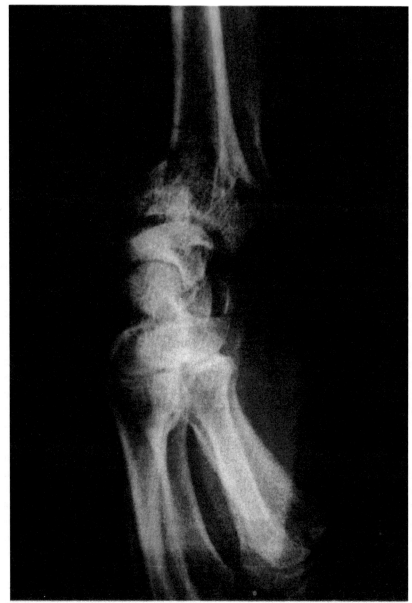

Figure 4.1a. Colles' fracture, lateral view.

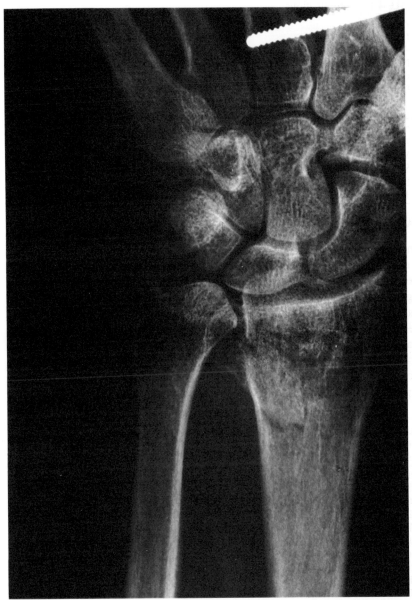

Figure 4.1b. Colles' fracture, anteroposterior after reduction and application of external fixator. Pin in upper part of film is part of external fixator used to distract fracture.

TABLE 4.1 Complications

Early
  Inadequate reduction
  Associated injury
  Nerve compression
  Edema
  Compartment syndrome
  Sympathetic dystrophy
Late
  Nerve compression
  Arthrosis
  Malunion
  Stiff hand
  Fixation problem
  Tendon rupture

CARPAL TUNNEL SYNDROME

Another common condition seen in the elderly is compression of the median nerve at the wrist, also known as carpal tunnel syndrome. Patients typically present with wrist and palm pain as well as numbness and tingling in the region innervated by the median nerve (thumb, index finger, middle finger and ulnar side of the ring finger). Paresthesias are often worse at night and frequently awaken patients. The unpleasant sensations may be relieved by shaking the hands or holding them under warm running water. Retrograde pain to the elbow or shoulder may be the predominant complaint. Patients often relate a recent history of weakness with inability to hold onto such objects as coffee cups or loss of dexterity with difficulty manipulating small objects. Although

TABLE 4.2 Classification of Calcium Pyrophosphate Crystal Deposition Disease[*]

Hereditary
  Slovakian
  Chilean
  Dutch
  French
  La Crosse
Sporadic (idiopathic)
Probable metabolic disease associations
  Hyperparathyroidism
  Hemochromatosis
  Hypothyroidism
  Gout
  Hypomagnesemia
  Hypophosphatasia
  Aging

[*] From Rodnan and Schumacher (28).

observed predominantly in women during the fifth and sixth decades, carpal tunnel syndrome occurs in elderly patients of both sexes. In this group, the symptoms often have an insidious onset and may be less well defined.

Physical examination often reveals diminished sensibility in the distribution of the median nerve (15,16), paresthesias on percussion over the median nerve at the wrist (Tinel's sign), numbness of the fingertips on prolonged flexion of the wrist (Phalen's test) and atrophy of the thenar musculature innervated by the median nerve (Figure 4.2A-C). Thenar atrophy is evidence of compression of the median nerve severe enough to warrant surgical release. Nonetheless, many elderly patients do not demonstrate the usual physical findings, thus making the diagnosis difficult.

Carpal tunnel syndrome is produced by increased pressure within the carpal canal. Although most cases are idiopathic, nonspecific flexor tenosynovitis is often found in patients undergoing surgical exploration. Local factors, such as major trauma, anomalous muscles or tumorous masses, have been implicated. In elderly patients, compression of the median nerve may be an early manifestation of rheumatoid arthritis, systemic lupus erythematosus, dermatomyositis, gout or chondrocalcinosis. Increased pressure in the canal can be due to the edema associated with hypothyroidism, or the local tissue may become infiltrated in patients with amyloidosis, sarcoidosis or leukemia (17,18). A strong association with stenosing tenosynovitis (trigger finger) has been noted. The examiner should carefully check patients with carpal tunnel syndrome for nodularity within the flexor tendons and actual or potential triggering.

One form of therapy is the use of resting splints in a neutral position to decrease pressure within the carpal canal. Such splints are particularly helpful in overcoming the tendency toward flexion of the wrist during sleep. The use of an oral nonsteroidal anti-inflammatory drug (NSAID) may also help relieve symptoms. Local injection of an anesthetic/corticosteroid mixture into the carpal canal but external to the median nerve in a patient with signs and symptoms of recent onset may afford good relief (19). Surgical intervention is indicated if there is persistence or recurrence of a disabling symptom (pain, paresthesia or weakness), thenar atrophy or marked loss of sensibility (20).

No long-term studies have been done to monitor the course of elderly patients after surgical decompression of the median nerve. In the authors' experience, most patients report prompt relief of pain. Recovery of sensibility and a decrease in paresthesias are less predictable results of therapy in elderly patients. Sensibility takes longer to return after surgical intervention in elderly than in young patients, and complete reversal of thenar atrophy rarely occurs.

STENOSING TENOSYNOVITIS

Limited motion of the thumb or fingers diagnosed as digital stenosing tenosynovitis, or "trigger finger," is the most common entity encountered in a hand-surgery office. It occurs most often in the dominant hand in women, with 75

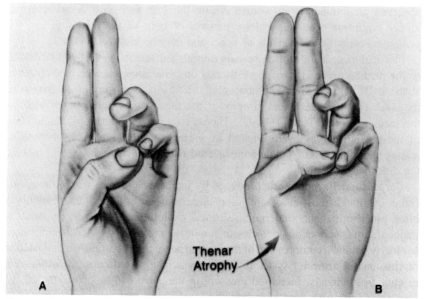

Figure 4.2a. Normal apposition of the thumb.

Figure 4.2b. Apposition with thenar atrophy.

percent of cases being in the middle or ring finger. Although the disease is usually considered idiopathic, the incidence is highest in patients with rheumatoid arthritis, myxedema or diabetes (18). Direct trauma or frequent repetitious hand movements, such as those associated with sewing or gardening, are contributing factors. Most patients describe inability to move the digit fully and may hear a popping sound on attempts at complete extension of the finger. Some elderly patients demonstrate locking in the extended position rather than in flexion. Local injection of an anesthetic/corticosteroid solution, within the tendon sheath but external to the tendon, is the usual initial management approach. If relief is not obtained after two or three injections, surgical release of the proximal portion of the fibro-osseous sheath is indicated. The expected result is unrestricted motion of the digit. However, for patients with degenerative arthritis at the distal joint or stiffness of the middle joint brought on by incomplete motion during medical management of the trigger finger, careful monitoring and a directed exercise program are required. Diabetic patients of any age can have a thickened tenosynovium, and their postoperative rehabilitation may be prolonged (18).

Another area commonly affected by stenosing tenosynovitis is the first extensor tendon compartment at the wrist (de Quervain's syndrome). The abductor pollicis longus and extensor pollicis brevis tendons pass through one or more sheaths at the radial styloid and are a common site of inflammation with subsequent synovitis and pain. This symptom complex may occur in elderly patients after

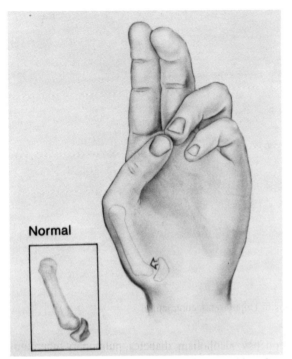

Normal

Figure 4.2c. With loss of thenar musculature, subluxation can develop at carpometacarpal joint.

a single episode of prolonged use. Injection of the sheath area with a corticosteroid preparation is the recommended initial therapy. Refractory cases may require surgical release of the sheaths of the first dorsal compartment with careful investigation for separate tendon tunnels and numerous tendon slips.

DUPUYTREN'S CONTRACTURE

This condition is usually asymptomatic and is manifested by a fibrous nodule in the palm at the base of the ring or little finger. With progression, a cordlike structure extends into the digit and draws the metacarpophalangeal and proximal interphalangeal joints into flexion (Figure 4.3). Although the etiologic basis of Dupuytren's contracture is uncertain, recent studies have related it to production of abnormal collagen (type III), probably on a genetic basis. Histologic studies show hypertrophy of the palmar fascia. Although the nerves and tendons may be entwined in the fibrous tissue, they are not primarily involved (21,22). A strong familial tendency exists, and the condition is more common among people of Northern European descent than in other populations. In one British population, 20 percent of the people over age 60 had evidence of Dupuytren's contracture (23). Other entities associated with Dupuytren's contracture (but not correlated

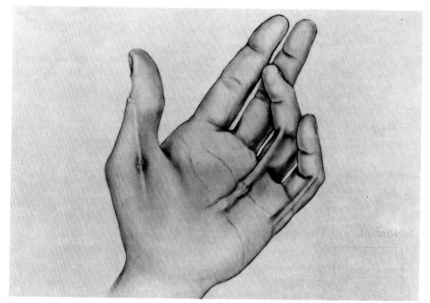

Figure 4.3. Fibrosis of tendons in Dupuytren's contracture.

with it statistically) include epilepsy, alcoholism, diabetes, pulmonary tuberculosis and chronic lung disease.

Although physical examination of many elderly patients demonstrates findings compatible with Dupuytren's contracture, surgical intervention may not be indicated. Specifically, excision of the palmar nodules and bands is contraindicated when there is no associated joint contracture. Patients are advised to return for reevaluation when they cannot place their hand flat on a surface like a tabletop (23). Minimum indications for surgical intervention include contracture of a metacarpophalangeal joint in excess of 30 degrees or measurable contracture of a proximal interphalangeal joint.

RHEUMATOID ARTHRITIS

The hands and wrists are often the initial site of involvement with rheumatoid arthritis. With progression of the disease, hand function may become seriously impaired. Although ulnar drift at a metacarpophalangeal joint is the lesion most commonly associated with rheumatoid arthritis, it is more the combined involvement of a number of small joints that can have a devastating effect on an elderly patient (24).

Rheumatoid arthritis commonly begins at an early age, but it can present in elderly patients. When the disease develops in later life, the degree of disability is often less than that seen in a young patient. A progressive course can be expected, nonetheless. The typical rheumatoid presentation of morning stiffness, symmetric bilateral pain and swelling of the small joints is rarely seen in elderly patients (25). The joints in the arm that are most frequently involved are the wrist and metacarpophalangeal joints. Extra-articular manifestations, such as nodules and arteritis, occur less often. Shoulder involvement is commonly seen and may be misdiagnosed as shoulder-hand syndrome. A complaint of bilateral shoulder and hand pain in an elderly patient should arouse suspicion of rheumatoid arthritis.

Mild ulnar drift at a metacarpophalangeal joint may be seen in an elderly patient who does not have inflammatory disease (21), and the diagnosis of rheumatoid arthritis must never be made by using this sign as the sole criterion. Care should be taken in diagnosing rheumatoid arthritis by laboratory means. The serum of elderly patients can have an increased concentration of rheumatoid factor and low titers of antinuclear antibodies. With advancing age, the incidence of these findings is even higher. Many elderly patients, especially those over age 70, have elevated erythrocyte sedimentation rates, and values of 50 to 60 are not uncommon in this population (25).

The surgical management of rheumatoid arthritis in elderly patients requires considerable judgment and expertise. The functional needs of a patient must be carefully weighed against the anticipated surgical outcome. Implant arthroplasty at the metacarpophalangeal joints should correct contractures and allow almost complete extension with a flexion arc of 55 to 75 degrees. Although relief of pain may be complete, restoration of grip strength is not. Patients with slowly progressive rheumatoid arthritis often have learned to function within the limits imposed on them. In the planning of a surgical approach, one strategy is to leave one hand capable of gripping small objects and reconstruct the other hand to allow full extension of the fingers to permit grasping large objects. In conclusion, any surgical procedure requires a thorough preoperative assessment as well as meticulous technique.

SERONEGATIVE ARTHROPATHIES

Joint disorders in the elderly that may be difficult to diagnose are the seronegative arthropathies. Although systemic lupus erythematousus is often considered a disease of young women, 12 percent of patients present after age 50 (26). Patients with lupus show fibrous and soft-tissue changes around the small joints of the hand. Roentgenograms may reveal joint subluxation or dislocation without erosion. The elbow frequently is spared. Lupus-likesyndromes can be produced by drugs often used by the elderly, such as procainamide, hydralazine and phenytoin (25,27).

During periods of remission, there is no sign of arthritis. About 20 to 30 percent of patients show progression of the disease, which in most cases eventually resemble rheumatoid arthritis. However, erosion of the bone rarely occurs. Together with the joint changes, there is muscle atrophy. Early in the course, one can see ulnar deviation of the digits. Interestingly enough, patients are able to correct this deviation over a relatively long period (Jacoud's phenomenon). In about 20 percent of patients, swan-neck and buttonhole deformities appear. Hyperextension of the thumb is another common phenomenon.

Psoriatic arthritis characteristically involves the distal interphalangeal joints. Nail involvement is seen in 80 percent of cases with discoloration, fragmentation, pitting and elevation of the distal portion of the nail (onycholysis). About 10 percent of patients with psoriasis show erosive arthritis. Roentgenograms often demonstrate gross destructive changes in isolated small joints, not unlike the changes seen in rheumatoid arthritis, as well as marked osteolysis, ankylosis and the "pencil-in-cup" appearance (28).

Patients with scleroderma often present with polyarthralgia and joint stiffness involving the fingers and wrist (29). Although appreciable warmth, redness and swelling of the digits are sometimes noted, the diffuse swelling is usually followed by gradual loss of subcutaneous tissue and typical "skeletonization" of the fingers (27). Roetgenograms demonstrate calcium deposits in the periarticular and soft tissues with resorption of the distal portions of the phalanges. Ulcers that show secondary infection should managed by close attention to local wound care and limited surgical intervention.

Scleroderma—Progressive Systemic Sclerosis

This uncommon disorder is characterized by inflammation of connective tissue in various organ systems. Pathologic changes in the vessels include thickening of the basement membrane and endothelium and, sometimes, a severe fibrotic process that results in a decrease in capillary blood flow. Most cases begin between ages 20 and 50, although the onset is occasionally at advanced age. Vasospasm is a common sign that appears as an intermittent Raynaud's phenomenon, or a sudden pallor or cyanosis of the fingers. When the disease progresses, fibrosis or obliterative endoarthritis can occur, leading to digital ulcers, necrosis and gangrene. Even at early stages, there are also typical microcirculatory changes at the nail folds.

GOUT AND PSEUDOGOUT

Crystal-Induced Diseases (See Table 4.2, p. 60.)

GOUT

There are two classical forms of gout:

1. Primary gout, in which the hyperuricemia is due to an inborn error of metabolism. This form is predominantly a disease of men; approximately 5 percent of cases are in women.
2. Secondary gout, in which the hyperuricemia is a consequence of an underlying disease or of treatment. This form also is mostly a disease of men, although about 25 percent of cases are in women.

Although the disease has a predilection for the joints of the legs, not uncommonly the joints of the arms are also involved. The disease most often has a polyarticular and asymmetric pattern. The initial attack often occurs in the fifth decade in men and after menopause in women although many patients do not show symptoms of the disease until after age 65. Gout often begins with a severely painful night attack; the joints are warm, red and extremely tender.

In the elbow, the most common sign is a warm, red, tender swelling of the soft tissue over the extensor surface that results from inflammation of the olecranon bursa. If left untreated the disease can cause extensive damage to the joint. Several years after the initial attack, tophi can be seen in the olecranon bursa.

Wrist and hand involvement is a common finding. All the compartments and tendon sheaths of the wrist may be involved. In the hand, the disease may involve the distal and proximal interphalangeal joints as well as the metacarpophalangeal joints. During an attack, the patient feels sick and occasionally has a fever and sweats. The course is variable. Without treatment, the attacks tend to occur more frequently and last longer. Later, the disease progresses into a chronic condition with persistent pain and deformity.

Tophi, deposits of monosodium urate crystals, are seen in the articular cartilage, subchondral bone, synovial membrane and joint capsules. In many cases, however, several years pass after the initial attack before such deposits can be demonstrated. In a case of long duration, the tophi may calcify or ossify. Roentgenograms characteristically show punched-out areas and cystic subchondral changes. Large areas of erosion are often seen as well.

More than 12 percent of patients have the first attack of gout after age 60. The diagnosis is established by the demonstration of strongly negative, birefringent, needle-shaped crystals in the involved joints. Within the hand and wrist, gouty tophi may resemble rheumatoid nodules and thus confuse the diagnosis. In general, tophi tend to be harder and more irregularly shaped than rheumatoid nodules, and they may become quite large. Uric acid deposits may account for trigger finger or carpal tunnel syndrome. Gouty attacks often occur after surgical procedures. Periarticular erythema and swelling may be mistakenly diagnosed as cellulitis or a septic joint when, in fact, the diagnosis is gout. This diagnostic confusion is especially common in elderly patients, who may not be able to give a clear history.

Even more than gout, pseudogout has a clear predilection for elderly patients, with most cases occurring after age 60. Roentgenograms demonstrate stippled or linear calcium deposits in the hyaline cartilage or fibrocartilage. Pseudogout represents a spectrum of diseases, ranging from acute, intermittent arthritis to chronic, persistent joint inflammation. Deposition of calcium within the cartilage is termed chondrocalcinosis (30). This arthropathy commonly involves joints in the arms that are not the primary sites of osteoarthritis, including the wrists, metacarpophalangeal joints, elbows and shoulders.

The roentgenographic appearance of chondrocalcinosis arthropathy in the hands is characteristic (31). Calcium deposits in the triangular fibrocartilaginous

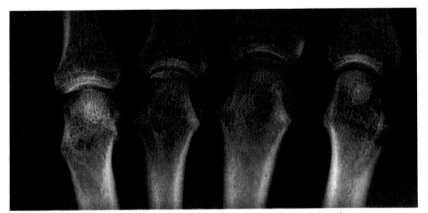

Figure 4.4. Arrows indicate sites of deposition of calcium pyrophosphate.

complex at the distal radioulnar joint and arthropathy of the second and third metacarpophalangeal joints are the most common abnormalities. Findings in the small joints include subchondral cysts, narrowing of the joint spaces and formation of osteophytes. As a result, the fingers may deviate and even demonstrate subluxation. Other roentgenographic findings are carpal cysts and calcium deposits around the metacarpophalangeal joints. The examiner should be aware that symptomatic involvement of a joint is not necessarily confirmed by roentgenographic evidence of calcium deposits (Figure 4.4).

Recently, calcium deposits within the cartilage have also been found to consist of dicalcium phosphate dihydrate, hydroxyapatite and calcium oxalate crystals (28). Apatite crystals have been demonstrated in osteoarthritic articular cartilage and in a high percentage of cases of osteoarthritic effusion. Apatite-deposition arthritis is associated with scleroderma, dermatomyositis and dialysis (28).

Other Rheumatic Disorders of the Hand and Wrist

Lars-Goran Larsson

POLYMYALGIA RHEUMATICA

A disease that is virtually limited to elderly patients (mean age, 65 to 70) is polymyalgia rheumatica. Most patients are women and they usually have symmetric shoulder stiffness. In occasional cases, there is soft-tissue swelling in the hands without joint redness or warmth (27). This low-grade synovitis can be difficult to differentiate from rheumatoid arthritis. Patients with polymyalgia rheumatica may also have Raynaud's phenomenon, which occurs secondary to giant-cell arteritis. An extremely high erythrocyte sedimentation rate is noted, and patients usually show a rapid response to corticosteroid therapy (26).

Many patients experience severe night pain and morning stiffness along with pain on motion. Arthralgia without joint swelling is a characteristic finding, and often the wrist and, occasionally, small joints of the hand are involved. Although the disease typically strikes large and medium-sized arteries, it occasionally affects the digital arteries as well.

SHOULDER-HAND SYNDROME

Patients with shoulder-hand syndrome commonly present with limitation of motion and pain in the shoulder as well as swelling stiffness and discomfort in the hand. With resolution of edema, further dystrophic changes in the hand may lead to the development of flexion contractures at the small joints. Ninety percent of patients with this syndrome are over age 50. Shoulder-hand syndrome is associated with a variety of underlying diseases, the most common being myocardial infarction, which precedes the syndrome in about 20 percent of cases (27). After the disease has run its course, more than 30 percent of patients are left with varying degrees of stiffness.

MISCELLANEOUS DISORDERS

Hemochromatosis

In this iron-storage disease, there is deposition of iron in parenchymal tissues as well as deposition of calcium pyrophosphate dehydrate crystals throughout the skeleton. Deposition of crystals may take place in the elbows, wrists and hands. Roentgenograms show narrowing of the joint spaces and formation of cysts and osteophytes. In the metacarpophalangeal joints, characteristic osteophytes, the so-called Bywaters hooks, develop. These changes are most often bilateral and symmetric.

Management consists of intra-articular injection of a corticosteroid, use of an NSAID in hemochromatosis and measures aimed at relief of symptoms.

Erythema Nodosum

This acute disorder is characterized by warm, bright red (later turning dark red), tender, nodular, cutaneous lesions of the lower portion of the legs. The condition can occur at any age, although the peak incidence is between ages 20 and 60. About 50 percent of patients suffer from arthritis. The female to male ratio of cases is 5:1. The disorder can occur as an allergic or a hypersensitivity reaction to a number of infectious diseases (tuberculosis, streptococcal infection, blastomycosis, cat-scratch fever, coccidioidomycosis, histoplasmosis, measles, lymphogranuloma venereum, leprosy, psittacosis) or drug usage. The condition can also develop in patients with ulcerative colitis, Crohn's disease, sarcoidosis, Behçet's syndrome or a malignant condition, such as lymphoma or leukemia. Soft-tissue swelling with or without effusion in the elbows, wrists and metacarpophalangeal and proximal interphalangeal joints is often noted. The pattern of these changes is mostly bilateral and symmetric. Patients report pain and morning stiffness. Fever often follows.

Diabetes Mellitus

A great variety of complications that increase in frequency with age occur in diabetics. In patients with severe diabetes of long duration, a true neuropathic (Charcot's) joint may develop with erosion and subluxation. This phenomenon may take place within the metacarpophalangeal joints and, sometimes (although rarely), the wrists.

Periarthritis of the hands sometimes occurs. Initially, patients report pain and stiffness. A diffuse swelling with warmth and redness sometimes follows. After time, the swelling subsides, with resultant atrophy of the skin and muscle. Many patients show contracture of the palmar fascia (Dupuytren's contracture). Other disorders which should complete your differential include Whipple's Disease and Bechet's Syndrome.

Amyloidosis

This disease results from infiltration by amyloid deposits. Any organ can be involved. Most cases occur between ages 50 and 60, but the disease can present in later life. Women and men are affected at the same frequency. There are five main types of amyloidosis

1. Primary (occurs without coexisting disease)
2. Secondary (associated with rheumatoid arthritis, inflammatory disease, multiple myeloma, neoplasm and other conditions)
3. Hereditary (cardiac involvement)
4. Senile (occurring at increased frequency with aging)
5. Localized tumors (in the respiratory tract).

Amyloid deposits may infiltrate into the synovium, capsule, bone, tendons and articular cartilage. Any joint in the body can be affected. The elbows are sometimes involved, but the disease more commonly affects the wrists and small joints of the hands. The clinical manifestations are bilateral polyarticular swelling, pain on motion, tenderness and limitation of motion. Amyloid deposits that resemble rheumatoid nodules may be seen. Morning stiffness is a common complaint.

Laboratory tests reveal an increased erythrocyte sedimentation rate as well as Bence Jones protein and synovial fluid of a noninflammatory type. The disease is diagnosed by biopsy of the synovium or stomach fat. The bone marrow contains a high concentration of plasma cells.

Roentgenograms reveal periarticular osteoporosis, erosion, subchrondosis, subluxation, lysis of bone, fractures and other changes that may eventually lead to destruction of the involved joints.

Management may be attempted with azathioprine or interferon. Relief of symptoms is also part of the management approach.

Carcinomatous Arthritis

This disease is often a seronegative arthritis (rheumatoid factor is rarely found) that resembles rheumatoid arthritis. The syndrome often indicates the possibility of a malignant lesion developing during the ensuing year. This condition rarely develops after a malignant disease, so it is not of metastatic origin. It can be associated with any malignant tumor, most often carcinoma of the lungs, breasts or prostate. Most cases occur around age 60; men are affected twice as often as are women. Usually the disease is asymmetric and polyarticular and characterized by pain and severe stiffness of sudden onset, often associated with fever and mental confusion. The response to NSAIDs is poor, and this observation, together with the systemic manifestations, distinguishes the disease from rheumatoid arthritis. Interestingly enough, palmar fasciitis and arthritis are encountered as associated conditions in elderly patients with tumors. Biopsy specimens from the joints show nonspecific synovitis. Surgical removal of the tumor may lead to dramatic resolution of the arthritis and other symptoms. Laboratory studies show an increased erythrocyte sedimentation rate.

Recognition and control of the malignant process are the clues to successful management.

Polymyositis, Dermatomyositis

These connective-tissue disorders of unknown origin are characterized by weakness of the proximal muscles. When polymyositis is accompanied by skin lesions, it is called dermatomyositis (about 25 percent of cases). The skin change is a diffuse erythema in the face (often with the pattern of butterfly rash), neck, upper arms and upper trunk. A red rash and edema of the eyelids (heliotropic) are other characteristic findings. Patients in whom dermatomyositis begins after age 50 have a high incidence of neoplasms (50 to 70 percent of cases). The disease occurs in all age groups, although most cases are in patients 45 to 55 years of age. The incidence is higher among blacks, in whom the peak age at onset is 55 to 64. The female to male ratio of cases is 2:1.

Clinical manifestations include muscle weakness (mostly of the shoulder girdle), weight loss, fever, joint pain with morning stiffness, Raynaud's phenomenon, dysphagia, bowel lesions and cardiomyopathy. Arthritis develops in about 40 percent of cases; in rare instances, it precedes the disease. In most cases, the pattern of involvement is bilateral and symmetric.

The fingers and wrists are usually involved; the elbows are occasionally affected. Physical examination shows warmth, redness and tenderness of the joints, often with effusion. There is severe pain, and restriction of motion may be a prominent finding. An interesting feature is dislocation of the interphalangeal joint of the thumb ("floppy-thumb sign").

Roentgenograms reveal periarticular osteoporosis, erosion, dislocation and calcium deposits.

Laboratory tests show an increased erythrocyte sedimentation rate and a high concentration of C-reactive protein. Rheumatoid factor is detected in half of the patients and antinuclear antibody in one-third. Electromyographic studies show an abnormal myographic pattern.

In elderly patients, there is a high degree of osteoporosis, so treatment presents a dilemma. It is customary to start with 40 mg of prednisolone and with a cytotoxic drug and to taper the dosage of prednisolone to a minimum of 10 mg (preferably 15 mg) daily. Other components of management include an NSAID and physical therapy to improve muscle strength. The physician should consider the possibility of a neoplasm in patients with dermatomyositis. Carcinoma is found most often, but melanoma, lymphoma and leukemia have been reported.

Tuberculosis

Tuberculosis is now an infrequent cause of tenosynovitis, but before the 1950s it was described relatively frequently. From time to time, cases are still reported, particularly among immigrants from developing countries, such as Mexico. Tuberculosis can also flare up during long-term cortisone therapy.

The flexor tendon sheaths of the fingers are most often affected. At this stage, patients are usually "worn out" because a focus often exists elsewhere in the body. Weight loss, slight fever and regional lymphadenopathy are common findings. The disease is diagnosed on the basis of demonstration of tubercle bacilli in the lesions by microscopy or culture. The tuberculin skin test almost always gives a positive result. Atypical mycobacteria, such as *Mycobacterium szulgai, M. kansasii, M. triviale* and *M. scrofulaceum,* have been discovered in rare cases.

Sarcoidosis is another unusual cause of tendinitis. Infrequent causes also include coccidiodomycosis and toxoplasmosis.

Management involves administration of a tuberculostatic drug. Kveim's test should be done if carcoid is suspected.

Fibrositis

This term is used to describe a number of ill-defined conditions in which pain, an aching sensation and stiffness are the main features. Although the "itis" in fibrositis indicates that such conditions are inflammatory, most are, in fact, not of this nature, so care must be employed in using this term. Its use should be restricted to describe soft-tissue pain and tenderness of viral and other infectious origin. Most cases considered as being fibrositis actually represent fibromyalgia syndrome. There are primary and secondary forms. The condition is deemed primary when there is no identifiable underlying cause; the condition is secondary when it has an underlying rheumatic or nonrheumatic cause (e.g., rheumatoid arthritis, osteoarthritis, systemic lupus erythematosus, hypothyroidism or trauma).

Primary fibromyalgia is encountered more often in women than in men; the female to male ratio of cases ranges from 5:1 to 10:1. Yunus and coworkers noted that the age of onset ranged from nine to 55 years and that the age at presentation ranged from 14 to 61 years with a mean of about 40 years. Hence, the primary cause is chronic rheumatic pain among young and middle-aged women.

Tenderness or trigger points are typically found in different locations including the upper border of trapezius, costochondral junctions, fatpad medial to the knee, over the intervertebral ligament, supraspinous muscles, upper outer quadrant of the buttock, about 1 inch distal to the origin of the extensor muscles to the hand and the lateral epicondyle.

Nonetheless, trigger points originate in only one location—the "tennis elbow" site. Numbness and tingling of the forearm, wrist and hand may result. Slight, diffuse swelling of the digit is sometimes noted.

For the diagnosis to be made, the tenderness must have existed at least three months and there must be at least four trigger points in at least three locations. Moreover, the results of laboratory tests must be within normal limits. In most cases, there also are sleep disturbances, with pain, stiffness and fatigue in the morning and weariness continuing throughout the day. Other criteria include chronic anxiety or tension, headache, irritable bowel syndrome and subjective complaints of swelling and numbness of the hands. Patients feel better during dry, warm weather and worse when it is cold and damp. Physical activity increases their sense of well-being.

It is not known why primary fibromyalgia syndrome is encountered relatively infrequently among elderly patients, although one explanation may be that they are under less occupational and emotional stress. Most elderly patients have experienced intermittent symptoms earlier in life, and with poorer sleep conditions, the syndrome starts. The death of the spouse occasionally triggers the syndrome.

Because most patients have a disturbance of stage 4, nonrapid eye movement, sleep, a nightime dose of a tricyclic antidepressant (amitriptyline, 25 mg or less) is usually helpful. Moderate physical activity, such as walking or swimming for 30 minutes per day at least five days per week, local application of heat, stretching and massage, also improves patients' sense of well-being and may afford a cure.

Carpal tunnel syndrome is frequently associated with "fibrositis syndrome." Six of the eight patients later suffered from inflammatory polyarthritis. Carpal tunnel syndrome may therefore be a manifestation of the underlying inflammatory disease and not a sign of fibrositis, which should be classified as secondary in those six patients. The possibility of preexisting diabetes must also be ruled out.

Eosinophilic Granulomatous Vasculitis (Churg-Strauss vasculitis)

This unusual form of vasculitis strikes small arteries and veins. The pathologic changes are necrotizing vasculitis and granuloma with infiltration by eosinophils. The etiologic basis of this condition is unknown. The mean age at onset is 50 years, but all age groups are affected. The female to male ratio of cases is 2:1. The main clinical features are respiratory abnormalities, fever and weight loss. There may also be cutaneous lesions and peripheral neuropathy.

Management involves the use of prednisolone at a high dosage (40 mg daily); a cytotoxic drug is often needed as well. The prednisolone should be tapered to a maintenance level (10 mg daily or less) when symptoms are under control.

Periarteritis Nodosa

This uncommon disorder can occur at any age but is encountered most often in elderly patients. The male to female ratio of cases is 2:1. This necrotizing vasculitis involves all layers of the medium-sized and small vessels. Also encountered are systemic manifestations, such as fever, weakness and weight loss. The vasa vasorum to the nerves are frequently involved, as manifested by peripheral neuropathy. Bruising occurs, and peripheral gangrene develops. In many cases, hypertension is also observed.

Laboratory studies shown an increased erythrocyte sedimentation rate, anemia, leukocytosis, thrombocytosis, proteinuria, hematuria and a high concentration of gamma globulins.

This disease is managed with prednisolone at a high dosage. In the acute stage, a cytotoxic drug is often needed as well. Methotrexate at a low dosage has given promising results. If left untreated the disease tends to be terminal, with patients surviving only a few months.

Wegener's Granulomatosis

This rare condition characterized by lesions of the nose is associated with systemic vasculitis. It can begin at any age, but most patients are between ages 22 and 55. Late in the course, endarteritis obliterans can occur in the digits.

Muscle cramps are occasionally troublesome to elderly patients. They usually develop in the hands after extreme muscle effort or at night. The cramps can be terminated by passive stretching, and they can be prevented somewhat by the application of heat (e.g., a hot bath) or the use of quinine sulfate (which lengthens the refractory period of muscles) or a drug that inhibits the activity of the spinal neurons (methocarbamol, Cyclobenzaprine, and diphenhydramine) (32).

There are many infrequent causes of joint pain in the hands and wrists of elderly patients. Septic arthritis is always a diagnostic consideration (27). Elderly patients with underlying chronic diseases are particularly susceptible to secondary joint sepsis from some other infection, such as pneumonia, bacterial endocarditis, urinary tract infection or osteomyelitis. Patients taking immunosuppressive agents or corticosteroids also are at increased risk. Other uncommon causes of arthropathy of the arms are abnormal thyroid or parathyroid function, acromegaly, dermatomyositis, periarteritis nodosa and malignant lesions. It is essential that the physician constantly reevaluate a patient and his or her response to therapy instead of continuing to rely on the original diagnostic impression if the patient is failing to respond to treatment as anticipated.

OSTEOARTHRITIS

Probably the most frequent cause of pain in the hands and wrists of elderly patients is osteoarthritis. This disease is so prevalent among the elderly that it is difficult to distinguish normal aging from degenerative joint disease (33). Disruption of the collagen fiber framework, a loss of proteoglycans and enzyme changes within the cartilage all diminish the ability of the joints to withstand stress (28,34). The most common site of involvement is the distal interphalangeal joints, resulting in hypertrophic and degenerative changes called Heberden's nodes. These nodes occur most frequently in women over age 50, and a strong hereditary tendency exists. This predisposition is obvious in about half of cases; many other cases are of traumatic origin. These joints are particularly susceptible to degenerative changes because of their small surface area in relation to the strong forces exerted on them at the points of insertion of the flexor digitorum profundus and terminal extensor tendons (35). Although Heberden's nodes are more closely associated with osteoarthritis, they may be seen in combination with rheumatoid arthritis (36).

Heberden's nodes are seen in occurrence with mucous cysts that resemble ganglia. The pain associated with mucous cysts may derive from the underlying degenerative joint disease or from tension on the skin. In long-standing cases, one may see grooving of the nail as well as angulation and collapse of the distal joints. If the overlying skin becomes attenuated, the cysts may rupture, causing intra-articular infection. Conservative management of mucous cysts consists of placement of a protected splint and oral administration of an NSAID or intra-articular injection of a corticosteroid (37). Even with such therapy recurrence is commonly observed.

Surgical intervention is rarely indicated in cases of degenerative disease of the distal joints because pain usually subsides after the inflammatory phase resolves. If there is collapse or marked angulation in association with persistent pain, arthrodesis may be required. Although technically feasible, implant arthroplasty of a distal joint is rarely indicated. Arthrodesis should result in a painless, stable, functional joint if the correct position is selected. Surgical management of mucous cysts involves resection of the synovial tissue in combination with excision of the dorsal osteophyte and debridement. Surgical management of inflamed distal joints occasionally leads to a flare-up.

Osteophytic enlargements in the proximal interphalangeal joints associated with degenerative joint disease are known as Bouchard's nodes. These nodular swellings are of familial origin and are most commonly seen in women after age 50. The joint enlargement is often associated with formation of Heberden's nodes as well. However, one does not typically see synovial cysts or severe angulation deformities, such as boutonnière or swan-neck deformities of the middle joints. With osteoarthritis, the primary problem is progressive stiffness of the proximal interphalangeal joints.

Degenerative disease of the proximal interphalangeal joints can be managed surgically by debridement, arthrodesis or arthroplasty. If a single large osteophyte is troublesome, excision of the hypertrophic bone and soft tissue may provide relief. Solid arthrodesis affords a painless, stable joint. However, immobility of the middle joint, particularly on the ulnar side, decreases dexterity and grip strength. Arthroplasty should provide an arc of motion between 15 and 75 degrees (38). However, the stability and longevity of implant arthroplasty are not yet known.

Erosive or inflammatory osteoarthritis occurs occasionally and is characterized by the abrupt, symmetric onset of pain and swelling in the small joints of the hands (39). The distal interphalangeal joints are primarily involved, although the proximal joints are sometimes affected as well. The typical patient is a woman about 50 years of age. The initial manifestations are a throbbing sensation in the fingertips, particularly at night, and engorgement of the pulp. When the painful synovitis subsides, nodular changes similar to those seen with primary osteoarthritis often remain. Instability of the mediolateral joints resulting in subluxation is observed. A small proportion of patients later suffer from classical rheumatoid arthritis.

Another part of the hand commonly affected by degenerative disease is the basal joint of the thumbs. This condition is seen most often in women in their fifties and sixties. In addition to primary arthritis of the trapeziometacarpal joints, (Figure 4.5) more than 50 percent of patients show osteoarthritic changes between the trapezium and the adjacent bones (trapezoid, scaphoid) (Figure 4.6). Such patients should be carefully examined for coexisting carpal tunnel syndrome. Conservative management consists of administration of an anti-inflam-

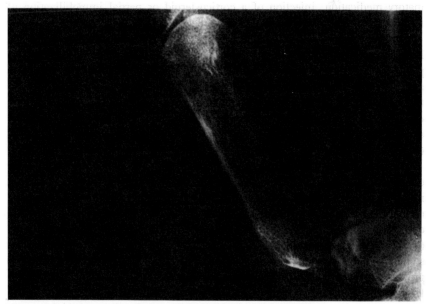

Figure 4.5. Degenerative disease of the basal joint of the thumb.

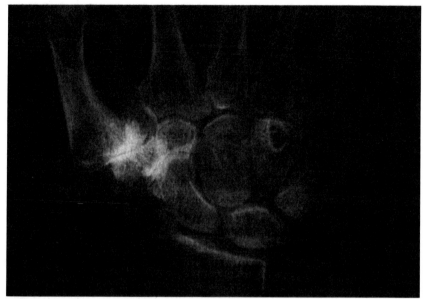

Figure 4.6. Severe osteoarthritic changes involving the trapezium, trapezoid and scaphoid bones.

matory medication, injection of a corticosteroid or partial immobilization of the thumb with a figure-of-eight splint.

Surgical options for the management of basal-joint arthritis include arthrodesis, hemiarthroplasy, a trapezium implant, fascial arthroplasty and total joint replacement. Arthrodesis is probably best suited for vigorous patients who anticipate placing heavy loads on their hands. If the arthritic changes are confined to the trapeziometacarpal joints, hemiarthroplasy or joint replacement can be considered. If there is pantrapezial arthritis, total resection is necessary and must be followed by a trapezial implant or fascial arthroplasy (Figures 4.7–4.8)

Although primary osteoarthritis of the radiocarpal or radioulnar joints is an unusual condition, post-traumatic changes that become symptomatic are not infrequently encountered in elderly patients (40). Watson and colleagues have recently described in detail the evolution of degenerative changes in the area of the wrist and have coined the term "scapha-lunate advanced collapse (SLAC)" (41,42). The earliest degenerative changes occur between the top of the radial styloid and the distal aspect of the scaphoid bones. Further alteration occurs proximally along the articular surface between the radius and scaphoid bones. However, degenerative changes then skip to the capitatolunate joint, sparing

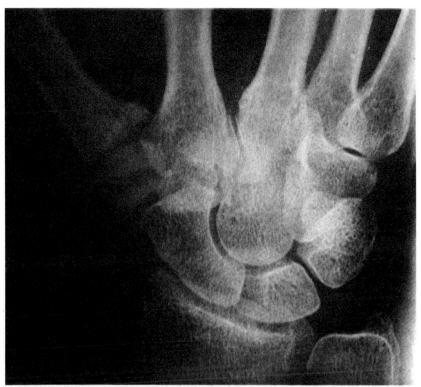

Figure 4.7. Silastic trapezoid implant used to manage arthritis of the carpometacarpal joint.

the radiolunate joint. The management approach for this collapse deformity proposed by Watson and colleagues is replacement of the scaphoid bone with an implant in combination with intercarpal fusion to transfer the forces to the unaffected radiolunate joint.

In summary, hand and wrist problems in elderly patients present difficult diagnostic and therapeutic challenges for primary-care physicians and their consultants. It may be difficult to establish a diagnosis because of the almost universal prevalence of degenerative joint disease in the elderly in combination with the numerous diseases that such patients can have. The specific needs of a patient must be carefully considered. One must always be aware of the tremendous tendency toward stiffness with any hand or wrist problem in elderly patients. Conservative management of generalized arthritic complaints often allows the patient to regain satisfactory function. The importance of the hands and wrists to the independence of elderly people must never be underestimated.

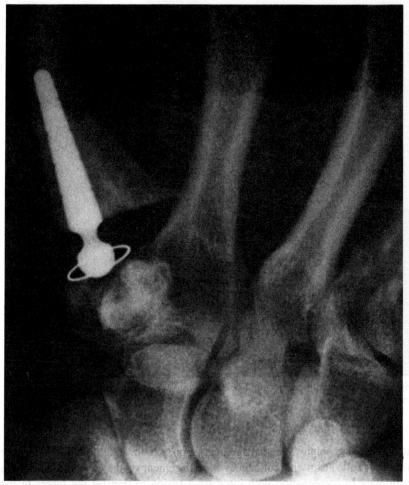

Figure 4.8. Cemented trapezial implant.

REFERENCES

1. Kolodny, A.L., and Klipper, A.R. Bone and joint diseases in the elderly. *Hosp. Pract.* 11:91–101, 1976.
2. Rossi, P., Fossaluzza, V., Pirrone, S., and Tosato, F. Flexion contractures and digital sclerosis in adult non-insulin-dependent diabetes. *Arthritis Rheum.* 27(8):960, 1984.
3. Wilson, R.L., and Liechty, B.W. Complications following small joint injuries. *Hand Clin.* 2(2):329–345, 1986.
4. Rowe, C.R. The management of fractures in elderly patients is different. *J. Bone Joint Surg.* 47A:1043–1059, 1965.
5. Salter, R.B. *Textbook of Disorders and Injuries of the Musculoskeletal System,* ed. 2. Baltimore, Williams & Wilkins, 1983.

6. Lincheid, R.L., Gartland, J.J., Jones, K.G., Grana, W.A., and Heppenstall, R.B. Symposium: Management of Colles' fractures. *Contemp. Orthop.* 8(2):123–144, 1984.

7. Lucas, G.L., and Sachtjen, K.M. An analysis of hand function in patients with Colles' fractures treated by rush rod fixation. *Clin. Orthop.* 155:172–197, 1981.

8. Cooney, W.P., Lincheid, R.L., and Dobyns, J.H. External pin fixation for unstable Colles' fractures. *J. Bone Joint. Surg.* 61A:840–845, 1979.

9. Nakata, R.Y., Chand, Y., Matiko, J.D., Frykman, G.K., and Wood, V.E. External fixators for wrist fractures: A biomechanical and clinical study. *J. Hand Surg.* 10A:845–851, 1985.

10. Bacorn, R.W., and Kurtzke, J.F. Colles' fracture: A study of 2,000 cases from the New York State Workmen's Compensation Board. *J. Bone Joint. Surg.* 35A:643–658, 1953.

11. Cooney, W.P., Dobyns, J.H., and Lincheid, R.L. Complications of Colles' fractures. *J. Bone Joint. Surg.* 62A:613–619, 1980.

12. Taleisnik, J., and Watson, H.K. Midcarpal instability caused by malunited fractures of the distal radius. *J. Hand Surg.* 9A:350–357, 1984.

13. Wilson, R.L., and Carter, M.S. Joint injuries in the hand: Preservation of proximal interphalangeal joint function, in Hunger, J.M., Schneider, L.H., Mackin, E.J., and Bell, J.A. (eds.): *Rehabilitation of the Hand.* St. Louis, Mosby, 1978, pp. 171–183.

14. Wilson, R.L., and Carter, M.S.: Management of hand fractures, in Hunter, J.M., Schneider, L.H., Mackin, E.J., and Bell, J.A. (eds.): *Rehabilitation of the Hand.* St. Louis, Mosby, 1978, pp. 154–183.

15. Silver, M.A., Gelberman, R.H., Gellman, H., and Rhoades, C.E. Carpal tunnel syndrome: Associated abnormalities in ulnar nerve function and the effect of carpal tunnel release on these abnormalities. *J. Hand Surg.* 10A:710–713, 1985.

16. Szabo, R.M., Gelberman, R.H., and Dimick, M.P. Sensibility testing in patients with carpal tunnel syndrome. *J. Bone Joint Surg.* 66A:60–64, 1984.

17. Dorwart, B.B. Carpal tunnel syndrome: A review. *Semin. Arthritis Rheum.* 14(2):134–140, 1984.

18. Gray, R.G., and Gottlieb, N.L. Rheumatic disorders associated with diabetes mellitus: Literature review. Semin. Arthritis Rheum. 6(1):19–34, 1976.

19. Green, D.P. Diagnostic and therapeutic value of carpal tunnel injection. *J. Hand Surg.* 9A:850–854, 1984.

20. Kulick, M.I., Kilgore, E.S., Jr., and Newmeyer, W.L. Long-term analysis of patients having surgical treatment for carpal tunnel syndrome. *J. Hand Surg.* 11A:59–66, 1986.

21. McFarlane, R.M. Patterns of the diseased fascia in the fingers in Dupuytren's contracture. Displacement of the neurovascular bundle. *Plast. Reconstr. Surg.* 54(1):31–44, 1974.

22. Skoog, T. The pathogenesis and etiology of Dupuytren's contracture. *Plast. Reconstr. Surg.* 31(3):258–267, 1963.

23. Hueston, J.T. Limited fasciectomy for Dupuytren's contracture. *Plast. Reconstr. Surg.* 27:569–585, 1961.

24. Wilson, R.L. Rheumatoid arthritis of the hand. *Orthop. Clin. North Amer.* 17:313–343, 1986.

25. Reich, M.L. Arthritis: Avoiding diagnostic pitfalls. *Geriatrics* 37(6):46–54, 1982.

26. Williams, T.F. (ed.). *Rehabilitation in the Aging*. New York, Raven Press, 1984, pp. 180–197.

27. Bienenstock, H., and Fernando, K.R. Arthritis in the elderly. An overview. *Med. Clin.* 60(6):1173–1189, 1976.

28. Rodnan, G.P., and Schumacher, H.R. (eds.). *Primer on the Rheumatic Diseases*, ed. 8. Atlanta, Arthritis Foundation, 1983.

29. Serup, J. Measurement of contractures of the digits in systemic sclerosis. *Dermatologica* 167:250–255, 1983.

30. Wilkins, E., Dieppe, P., Maddison, P., and Evison, G. Osteoarthritis and articular chondrocalcinosis in the elderly. *Ann. Rheum. Dis.* 42:280–284, 1983.

31. Bourqui, M., Vischer, T.L., Stasse, P., Docquier, C., and Fallet, G.H. Pyrophosphate arthropathy in the carpal and metacarpophalangeal joints. *Ann. Rheum. Dis.* 42:626–630, 1983.

32. Grob, D. Common disorders of muscles in the aged, in Reichel, W. (ed.): *Clinical Aspects of Aging*. Baltimore, Williams & Wilkins, 1983, pp. 329–343.

33. Moskowitz, R.W., Howell, D.S., Goldberg, V.M., and Mankin, H.J. *Osteoarthritis: Diagnosis and Management*. Philadelphia, Saunders, 1984.

34. Akeson, W.H., and Gershuni, D.H. Articular cartilage physiology and metabolism in health and disease, in Resnick, D., and Niwayama, G. (eds.): 2 Philadelphia, Saunders, 1981.

35. Radin, E.L., Parker, H.G., and Paul, I.L. Pattern of degenerative arthritis. Preferential involvement of distal finger joints. *Lancet*: 377–379, 1971.

36. Campion, G., Dieppe, P., and Watt, I. Heberden's nodes in osteoarthritis and rheumatoid arthritis. *Brit. Med. J.* 28:1512, 1962.

37. Friedman, D.M., and Moore, M.E. The efficacy of intraarticular steroids in osteoarthritis: A double-blind study. *J. Rheum.* 7(6):850–856, 1980.

38. Dryer, R.F., Blair, W.F., Shurr, D.G., and Buckwalter, J.A. Proximal interphalangeal joint arthroplasty. *Clin. Orthop.* 185:187–194, 1984.

39. Ehrlich, G.E. Inflammatory osteoarthritis—I. The clinical syndrome. *J. Chronic Dis.* 25:317–328, 1972.

40. Chernin, M.H., and Pitt, M.J. Radiographic disease patterns at the carpus. *Clin. Orthop.* 187:72–80, 1984.

41. Watson, H.K., and Brenner, L.H. Degenerative disorders of the wrist. *J. Hand Surg.* 10A(6): 1002–1006, 1985.

42. Watson, H.K., and Ballet, F.L. The SLAC wrist: Scapholunate advanced collapse pattern of degenerative arthritis. *J. Hand Surg.* 9A(3):358–365, 1984.

Chapter 5

Robert G. Volz
Robert R. Karpman

Hip

Hip problems are commonly encountered in the elderly. In the later decades, degenerative processes exhibit an affinity for the hips, and the pelvis and hips become major sites of primary bone disease and metastases. Because of the increased occurrence of falls with aging, these regions are also subject to much trauma and more frequent fractures. For these reasons, knowledge of anatomic structures and the physical examination are especially important to physicians who care for elderly patients.

Evaluation of any hip problem begins with a thorough history of the presenting complaint. The pattern of hip pain is important diagnostic information. The components of the pattern are the anatomic area of involvement and the factors relating to onset or aggravation. For instance, pain in the area of the greater trochanter and the lateral aspect of the thigh suggests inflammation of the trochanteric bursa or entrapment of the lateral cutaneous nerve of the femur. Noteworthy findings in the differential diagnosis include hypoesthesia, hyperesthesia and aggravation of pain while lying on the side, crossing the leg or walking or climbing stairs. The latter findings are associated with bursitis, the former with pressure on the nerve. Pain that arises from the acetabulum may be referred to the buttock, groin or, more commonly, distally along the front of the thigh to an area just above the knee. In children and, less frequently, in adults, hip pain may be mistakenly thought to arise from the knee. Pain confined to the inner aspect of the thigh is more commonly associated with thrombophlebitis or cellulitis. Inguinal and femoral herniation must also be included in the differential diagnosis. In rare instances, undiagnosed diabetes mellitus presents as femoral neuritis, as do malignant lesions of the upper lumbar vertebrae with associated radiculopathy.

Perhaps the most common source of confusion over the origin of pain involves radicular pain, which arises from the spinal nerve roots. In general, pain confined to a buttock is of radicular origin and does not originate, from the hip. Further help in the differentiation between pain of radicular origin and true hip pain is a description of pain extending down the posterior aspect of the thigh and especially the calf; this pattern being further evidence of radiculopathy. Differentiation between these two sources of pain is discussed in greater detail later in relation to the physical examination.

Another important point in the differential diagnosis of pain is the distinction between pain at rest and pain that occurs with use of the hip, in static or dynamic loading situations. Pain at rest suggests a pathologic process, such as tumor, infection or inflammation. Pain that occurs with weight-bearing activity or movement is mechanical in nature and more likely of arthritic origin. Patients with arthritic pain typically report nearly complete relief at rest but a progressive increase in pain with movement, particularly weight-bearing activity. These easily determined patterns of hip pain provide insights concerning the likely anatomic or pathologic source of the complaint.

PHYSICAL EXAMINATION

The physical examination should include a careful assessment of gait, an evaluation of active and passive ranges of motion, a determination of hip muscle strength and a measurement of any discrepancy in leg length.

Analyzing abnormalities of gait requires careful observation and appreciation of normal gait. Because there are so many aspects of normal gait, a systematic approach is essential. First, one should observe separately the various anatomic components that comprise gait: torso posture, hip mechanics (motion and posture), knee mechanics (motion and alignment) and ankle and foot mechanics (alignment and step off). In addition, the time spent on each supporting foot should be noted, as should the stride of each advancing leg.

Many patients with an abnormality of gait secondary to hip pain walk in the following manner: The torso lurches toward the painful side. If both hips are painful, the torso lurches to the weight-bearing side with each step. In displacing the torso toward the weight-bearing side, the patient is attempting to lessen the load on the painful hip by placing more of the body weight on the supporting leg. This maneuver shortens the lever effect of the weight of the torso on the supporting hip, thereby lessening the load on the head of the femur. The posture of the torso in relation to the supporting leg should also be noted. Painful, arthritic hips provoke a flexion contracture, which is readily identified by a stooped posture.

Next, the arc of motion of the advancing hip should be noted. Normally, there are about 30 to 35 degrees of motion in a normal gait. With arthritic change or hip pain, the arc of motion may be diminished or eliminated. As weight is borne on each advancing leg, a small arc of pelvic rotation takes place, and there is a slightly increased varus alignment of the weight-bearing leg. With practice, the examiner can identify each parameter of gait and become proficient in the assessment of hip problems.

Assessment of knee mechanics often aids in the recognition of a fixed hip deformity. For example, a flexion contracture at the hip will not provide for sufficient hip extension to permit complete extension of the knee as weight is brought over the supporting leg. Thus, the examiner must consider the hip as a potential source of a flexion contracture at the knee. The identification of such a contracture is important if surgical intervention is being considered for the management of hip disease. If an appreciable flexion contracture at the knee persists postoperatively, it will not be possible to bring the hip joint into complete extension, while supine or standing. In this regard, a fixed equinus deformity at the ankle would also prevent complete extension of the knee and hip, thus giving rise to the same difficulty in achieving satisfactory surgical correction of a hip flexion deformity.

Perhaps at this juncture, we should consider the issue of the clinical implications of a fixed flexion contracture at the hip. The alignment of the legs is critical to the issue of expenditure of energy with standing and walking. When the knee and hip are extended in the standing position, little energy is required to produce muscle contraction to sustain the torso in an upright posture over the supporting leg because the center of gravity falls posterior to the hip and anterior to the knee. Little muscle contraction is required to maintain a standing posture because the hip and knee are "locked" into full extension. The moment the torso is placed in flexion over the supporting leg, the hip extensors require greater energy to maintain the torso upright. In addition, the center of gravity of the torso, which lies immediately in front of the second sacral segment, now acts on the hip with increased leverage, thereby increasing the stress on the hip. If there has been an arthritic change in the hip, the end result is increased discomfort because arthritic pain is a function of stress per surface area.

Other aspects of gait should be assessed, including the length of time that weight is borne on each foot. When pain occurs with weight-bearing activity, the patient quickly unweights the painful side by advancing the nonpainful, supporting leg more quickly. Thus, the time weight is borne on each leg is unequal, being noticeably shorter on the painful side. This alteration is only one of several patterns seen with an antalgic gait. Normally, in the course of walking, the unweighted side of the pelvis is elevated slightly to facilitate advancement of the unweighted leg. When there is weakness of the short abductor muscles of the hip, a lurching gait is observed, wherein the unweighted side of the pelvis falls toward the ground. This gait pattern, the Trendelenburg gait, may also be observed when the head of the femur lacks stability within the acetabulum. A good example is congenital dislocation of the hip, in which proximal slippage occurs with weight-bearing activity.

A third aspect of gait is the stride of each advancing leg. A flexion contracture at the hip or knee or an appreciable loss of motion in either joint results in a shorter stride on the involved side. After gait has been carefully evaluated, the active and passive ranges of motion should be assessed. The arc of active motion identifies what a patient is capable of with active muscle control, a situation that increases the stress on a joint. The arc of passive motion is the true extent of motion available at the hip. Frequently, the true extent of motion cannot be determined until a patient has obtained sufficient relief of pain from an analgesic or anesthetic.

Much can be learned by merely observing a patient as he or she sits while the history is being obtained. Many patients with hip pain do not cross the involved leg or acutely flex the painful hip. With the patient sitting and the knee and hip flexed at right angles, the examiner can make a first assessment of the relative lengths of the leg and thigh. Shortening of the thigh suggests an adduction contracture or intrinsic shortening of the femur. Aseptic necrosis of the head of the femur, intrinsic shortening of its shaft due to malunion and a growth arrest problem are only three of the many possibilities to be considered. The arcs of internal and external rotation can also easily be determined in the sitting position. Almost without exception, internal rotation is the first plane of motion lost with any intrinsic abnormality of the hip because of the proximity of the external rotators of the hip, which become spastic with hip disease. Pain associated with rotation of the hip also is a sine qua non of an intrinsic abnormality of the hip. This pain must be distinguished from the pain that occurs with a straight leg-raising maneuver, which may be of radicular origin.

The planes of motion that should be recorded are abduction/adduction, internal/external rotation and flexion/extension. Extension and abduction of the hip are frequently diminished with any painful hip problem. If motion is limited for a sufficiently long period, a permanent contracture of the hip capsule and adjacent musculature will occur. In most cases, there is an adequate arc of flexion because the sitting position generally occupies a large part of one's day. With the patient in the supine position, one cannot determine whether there has been a loss of extension of the hip because of the ability of the pelvis to hyperextend on the lumbar spine. To determine whether a loss of extension has occurred, the examiner must hyperflex the opposite hip to flex the pelvis in relation to the lumbar spine. If the painful hip assumes a posture of flexion that cannot be reversed by forced extension of the thigh, a fixed flexion contracture exists. In general, if internal rotation is the first plane of motion limited by a hip problem, extension will be the second plane of involvement.

Information can often be gained by palpating the bony landmarks surrounding the pelvis and hip. An imaginary line drawn from the anterior superior spine to the ischial tuberosity should transect the greater trochanter. In cases of fracture or congenital dislocation of the hip, the trochanter lies above this line (Nélaton's line). The examination should be done with the patient lying on the side and having the upside hip in adduction. Palpation over the greater trochanter that elicits pain suggests trochanteric bursitis. Painful dysesthesia over the lateral and proximal aspects of the thigh suggests entrapment of the lateral cutaneous nerve (meralgia paresthetica). Palpation slightly medial to the anterior superior spine along Poupart's (inguinal) ligament may reproduce this symptom.

In cases of acute trauma, alignment of the leg is of considerable importance. Acute traumatic dislocation of the hip is manifested by characteristic deformities. With an anterior dislocation, the leg is externally rotated and extended. By contrast, with a posterior dislocation, there is internal rotation, adduction and slight flexion. A displaced fracture of the hip also is manifested by a predictable deformity, an externally rotated and shortened leg. Any attempt at passive rotation of the hip provokes pain. Fractures of the pubic rami are also common occurrences in the elderly. Physical examination may be helpful in differentiating between this type of fracture and a fracture of the hip or femur. A fracture of the pubic rami does not give rise to a deformity of the leg, but gentle attempts to passively abduct the leg on the pelvis produce pain in the groin. Gentle attempts to rotate the thigh on the pelvis usually provoke pain only if a hip has been fractured.

Auscultation of a painful pelvis after a fall also frequently helps in determining whether a fracture has been sustained, even if there is no discernible deformity. The principle of this part of the examination is the conduction of sound waves along an unbroken, solid medium as opposed to an interrupted one. The diaphragm of a stethoscope is placed against the symphysis pubis and the index finger palpates firmly over the midportion of the patella. If the femur or a pubic ramus has been fractured, transmission of sound waves will be disrupted on the involved side and the pitch of the sound will be lower on the involved side than on the uninvolved side.

The occasional dilemma of distinguishing pain in the hip due to a back problem from that due to a hip problem can frequently be resolved expeditiously by injecting a local anesthetic into the hip joint. If the pain arises from an intra-articular source, it will quickly be elminated by this maneuver. If the pain is unaffected, it must be radiating from a source outside the joint capsule. Aspiration or injection of the hip is most easily performed in the supine position. The landmarks for insertion of the needle, usually an 18- or 20-guage spinal needle, are the greater trochanter, anterior superior spine and tip of the superior pubic ramus. The head of the femur lies in a plane level with the greater trochanter and at the junction of the inner and middle thirds of a line drawn from the pubic ramus to the anterior superior spine. The needle is placed properly within the joint space if it passes through the thick, resistant capsule and strikes the neck or head of the femur.

Normally, a scant amount of synovial fluid is contained within the joint. Spontaneous filling of the syringe is a sign of an abnormal fluid collection. Fluid aspirated from the hip should be sent for an analysis of sugar content, examination for crystals by microscopy under polarized light and cell and differential cell counts. If infection is suspected, the fluid should be sent to the laboratory in the aspiration syringe and cultured as quickly as possible on aerobic and anaerobic mediums.

RADIOGRAPHIC EXAMINATION

An essential part of any evaluation of pain in the pelvis or hip is a radiographic examination. Some general guidelines in the assessment of routine films will now be presented.

The quality of bone observed on a radiograph is important because osteoporosis is a common accompaniment of aging, especially in women and bedridden patients. Only a rough assessment of the degree of mineral loss is possible with routine films. A loss of mineral content becomes discernible only when 30 to 40 percent of the mineral has disappeared. More precise documentation of mineral content is possible with the dual-photon emission technique. Care should also be taken to identify focal areas of bone loss or destruction, a finding that in many cases is subtle.

A common error is to focus on the central area of a film, overlooking the periphery, or corners, where less obvious but important findings may exist. The quality of bone loss and the body's response offer helpful insights regarding the differential diagnosis. The slower the process, the greater the opportunity for the body to respond by creating a reactive bony sclerosis. Because many primary tumors of bone have the potential to form bone, special attention should be focused on the density of a lesion. Metastatic lesions do not possess this capability.

In any radiographic evaluation of the pelvis, an assessment of the width of the joint space is a basic consideration. With inflammatory types of arthritic change, a symmetric narrowing is noted, whereas with degenerative types, the abnormality is focal. The width of the supporting acetabular subchondral plate, the sorrel, is a reflection of the load transmitted by the head of the femur to the acetabulum. With a degenerative change in the head of the femur and a loss of cartilage over the dome of the hip joint, the width of the sclerotic plate frequently becomes narrowed. There is also a fairly constant relationship of the head of the femur to the medial wall of the acetabulum. The width of the medial joint space should be between 10 and 15 mm. With an inflammatory change that results in a loss of cartilage, this distance narrows as the head of the femur begins to migrate, or protrude, into the pelvis. In cases of osteoarthritis in which loss of cartilage is focal and superior (mostly around the rim of the acetabulum), the head of the femur subluxes, thus widening the medial joint space.

Recognition of undisplaced fractures, especially in the elderly, is often difficult, and repeat films several weeks apart are frequently required. The best method for identifying such elusive fractures is to follow the outline of each cortical shadow, looking carefully for any suggestion of cortical disruption. Lastly, Paget's disease is a common asymptomatic condition in elderly patients, and it can be identified by a loss of clearly defined trabecular bone, fuzziness of cortical shadows and an increase in the bony dimensions of the area of involvement.

Attention will now be turned to several commonly observed diseases of the pelvis and hip joints in the elderly.

OSTEONECROSIS OF THE HEAD OF THE FEMUR

The first symptom of osteonecrosis of the hip is pain at rest and with weight-bearing activity. Radiography is not helpful in identifying this process at an early stage. Magnetic resonance imaging, a newer technique that is extremely useful in this regard, is the procedure of choice. As the osteonecrosis progresses to involve more of the head of the femur, radiographic changes become apparent. Findings include sclerosis and lysis of bone just beneath the subchondral plate of the head of the femur and, later, separation of subchondral cancellous bone from the plate, as viewed in the lateral projection of the hip joint. The latter finding is perhaps the most unequivocal early change seen on radiographs. By the time this change is apparent, weight-bearing activity is compromised, often necessitating the use of a walking aid. The examiner should be aware that in approximately 10 percent of cases, the process is bilateral.

Although the cause of osteonecrosis of the hip often remains obscure, it is known to result from alcohol abuse, use of corticosteroids, hemoglobinopathies, a history of prior trauma (in elderly patients, especially an intracapsular fracture or a dislocation of the hip), hyperuricemia, systemic lupus erythematosus, a history of irradiation of the area of involvement and inflitrative lesions, including metastatic tumors. Evidence of increased bone marrow pressure and altered venous drainage has been observed in all stages of the disease. Management of osteonecrosis has been disappointing because it has not been possible to slow down appreciably the progressive loss of articular cartilage and subchondral bone collapse. Orthopedic reconstructive procedures, such as osteotomy of the proximal aspect of the femur or placement of a prothesis, are eventually considered in most cases.

Another condition not infrequently observed in the elderly is Paget's disease. In this focal disorder, the normal trabecular architectrue is replaced by a weaker, disorganized lamellar bone. If the area of involvement is one where appreciable stress occurs, a deformity frequently arises and becomes progressive. It has been estimated that between 1 and 3 percent of people over age 45, particularly men, have Paget's disease, especially of the hip and pelvis. The recent identification of intranuclear inclusion bodies and adjacent osteoclasts has given rise to speculation that Paget's disease is of viral origin. Because the disease is most commonly asymptomatic, it is usually recognized as an incidental finding on radiographs. However, a small proportion of patients present with pain.

Further confirmation of the diagnosis includes an elevated serum titer of alkaline phosphatase and increased urinary excretion of hydroxyproline. Therapy is usually reserved for patients with symptoms and those with progressive deformity of sufficient magnitude to compromise function or predispose to a fracture.

Management approaches include subcutaneous administration of synthetic salmon calcitonin and oral use of disodium etidronate, a diphosphonate compound that is taken at a dosage of 5 mg per kilogram per day for no longer than six months. Longer-term therapy places patients at risk for osteomalacia. Mithramycin is also effective, although it probably should be used only in patients with severe disease in whom a rapid response is desired and in patients who have not responded to other therapy.

OSTEOARTHRITIS

Osteoarthritis is probably the most common cause of hip problems in elderly patients. The diagnosis and medical management of this disease have been discussed previously in this and other chapters; however, certain aspects of management should be emphasized here, particularly the use of assistive devices. When recommending use of a cane, it is important to tell a patient that the device should be used on the side *opposite* the involved hip to decrease the stress on that hip. Most patients mistakenly use assistive devices on the involved side. In addition, patients with osteoarthritis who undergo total hip replacement have an increased incidence of heterotopic bone development postoperatively. This phenomenon leads to increased stiffness and severe debility and should be managed with a diphosphonate (20 mg per kilogram per day) during the perioperative and postoperative periods or with a course of low-dose radiation therapy (1000 to 2000 rads) directed to the involved hip.

Diseases associated with the formation of heterotopic bone after total hip replacement also include ankylosing spondylitis and post-traumatic arthritis.

Other arthritic conditions of the hip that should be considered in elderly patients are rheumatoid arthritis, ankylosing spondylitis, pigmented villonodular synovitis, traumatic arthritis and arthritis secondary to avascular necrosis. These diseases can be easily diagnosed on the basis of the history, physical examination and radiographic findings.

Even though septic arthritis is less commonly seen in the hip than in other joints, it should be considered in patients with hip pain of sudden onset, particularly if they are immunocompromised. Chronic granulomatous infection, such as tuberculosis, begins less abruptly, and the diagnosis is often difficult. Aspiration of the hip, biopsy of the synovium in patients with chronic infection and debridement should be performed to spare the articular surface.

TOTAL HIP REPLACEMENT

This surgical procedure has had a major impact on the management of arthritis, particularly in elderly patients. Arthroplasty creates a painless hip, allowing for increased mobility and independence in activities of daily living. Morbidity associated with total hip replacement includes infection, pneumonia and increased deep-vein thrombosis. These complications are not increased among elderly patients as compared to younger patients undergoing a similar procedure.

Pulmonary embolism secondary to deep-vein thrombosis is still an important and difficult-to-prevent complication of total hip replacement. The diagnosis may not be made until the patient complains of pleuritic chest pain. In many cases, there is no swelling of the involved limb or tenderness in the calf. The most direct technique for making the diagnosis is venography, which demonstrates obstruction of the pelvic veins, but not always on the involved side. Many articles have described prophylaxis for deep-vein thrombosis (1–5); warfarin, heparin, aspirin and other agents have been tried, all with mixed results. The procedure of choice at this writing is the use of adjusted subcutaneous doses of heparin to keep the partial prothrombin time slightly above normal. A recent study (6) has demonstrated that the incidence of pulmonary embolism and deep-vein thrombosis are decreased in patients treated with this regimen.

Late complications of total hip replacement include septic or aseptic loosening of the prosthesis. In either case, there is a progressive increase in pain in the operated hip. The pain usually resolves with "loading" of the prosthesis: Rising from bed or a chair aggravates the pain, and a short period of ambulation relieves it by allowing the prosthesis to settle in the femoral canal.

Physical examination may demonstrate loss of motion, a pronounced limp or pain on pistoning of the hip. Radiographs show increased lucency around the bone-cement interface. There may be an area of sclerosis around the cement. The white cell count is normal or slightly elevated, but the erythrocyte sedimentation rate in cases of septic loosening is frequently elevated.

It may be difficult to determine whether loosening of a prosthesis is related to infection. Aspiration of the hip and biopsy of tissue from the bone-cement interface is helpful. Septic loosening is most often caused by staphylococci, although Gram-negative organisms may be responsible in severe cases.

Management of septic loosening depends on the offending organism. In cases due to *Staphylococcus epidermidis,* removal of the prosthesis, debridement of the tissue and immediate revision with an antibiotic-impregnated cement is a feasible approach. In severe cases, removal of the prosthesis, debridement and implantation of antibiotic beads that provide an increased local concentration of the drug may be tried; revision is performed six to 12 weeks later. Success rates for reoperation are markedly lower than the rates for initial joint replacement. Nonetheless, acceptable results, particularly in cases of aseptic loosening or mild infection, can be anticipated.

A late complication that occurred in the past was breakage of the prosthesis, particularly the femoral stem. This problem has been eliminated by the use of better-designed prostheses made of stronger metals.

Fractures below the prosthesis, especially in osteoporotic bone, present a difficult problem. Such fractures have been managed by bedrest in traction, internal fixation with plates and screws and, in many cases, revision with a prosthesis having a longer stem. The managment approach depends on the site and type of fracture.

It should be mentioned here that many patients who undergo total hip replacement with a "cementless" type of prosthesis experience thigh pain for four to six months. This pain appears to be related to acute changes in the stress within the femoral canal. Reassurance should be given that this pain is not unexpected and will disappear over time.

OSTEOPOROSIS AND HIP FRACTURES

It is important to recognize that bone is not a static tissue but one that is in a constant state of flux, continually being formed and resorbed. This constant activity is performed by bone-forming cells (osteoblasts) and bone-resorbing cells (osteoclasts) on the collagen, which serves as a scaffolding for the laying down of hydroxyapatite, the major mineral in bone. Although the turnover rate and cell function of bone may be slightly decreased with age, bone healing occurs at approximately the same rate in people of all ages, unless there are extenuating circumstances, such as metastatic disease, poor nutrition, infection or immunosuppression.

Why, then, are fractures so common in the elderly? The answer is related to one important factor—bone mass—which decreases dramatically as the aging process continues.

Bone mass can be defined as the total amount of bone in the body at any point in time. There are constant changes in bone mass relating to its turnover rate. Bone mass increases at a steady rate until it reaches a maximum at age 30. In the ensuing years, bone mass declines at a rate of approximately 0.5 to 1 percent per year. After menopause, bone mass is lost at a substantially increased rate, leading to osteoporosis and fractures. It has been estimated that in the early postmenopausal period, 2 to 5 percent of bone mass is lost each year. By ages 75 to 80, however, bone mass in men and women is approximately, the same. It has been reported that when bone mass reaches a critical level, there is a 75 to 80 percent risk for fractures secondary to an appreciable decrease in structural strength. Minimal or even no trauma can lead to fracture formation. This loss in bone mass is commonly referred to as osteopenia.

When a fracture has developed secondary to osteopenia, the clinical syndrome of osteoporosis exists. Approximately 40 to 50 percent of American women over age 50 have osteoporosis, which contributes to more than 175,000 hip fractures per year and a greater number of fractures in the vertebral bodies, wrists and shoulders. These fractures obviously create substantial health-care expenditures. It has been estimated that approximately $3 billion are spent annually treating patients with hip fractures. There are several risk factors in the development of osteoporosis, including prolonged use of cortico-steroids, parathyroid and thyroid disorders, poor nutrition (i.e., inadequate dietary calcium), intake of caffeine, consumption of alcohol and smoking. However, the most common form of the disease is "senile," or postmenopausal, osteoporosis, the etiologic basis of which remains obscure. It is believed that the rapid decrease in estrogen levels that occurs after menopause has a destabilizing effect on bone, leading to increased resorption. This effect may be related to calcitonin, a hormone produced by the thyroid gland. To date, there are few methods for increasing bone mass once osteoporosis has developed. However, there are several methods for stabilizing bone mass or preventing the decrease in bone mass that normally precedes menopause. In addition, the structural strength of bone can be further decreased by inadequate intake of vitamin D, which leads to osteomalacia. This mechanism is particularly prevalent among the elderly, who are unable to be outside in ultraviolet light, particularly those who are institutionalized.

Osteoporosis is diagnosed after an overt fracture or on a routine radiograph of the chest in which thinning of the vertebral bodies is noted. This thinning often leads to the so-called codfish vertebrae described in radiology textbooks. However, 40 percent of the bone mass has been lost before any radiographic change is apparent. Other, more sensitive methods of diagnosing osteopenia include single- and dual-photon densitometry and quantitative computerized axial tomography. The accuracy of dual-photon densitometry and quantitative CAT is approximately equal, with a 2 to 3 percent variance in measurements. Measurements should be obtained approximately every six to 12 months to determine the rate of bone loss. Single measurements alone do not enable a physician to determine the rate of bone loss and, again, it is the *rate* of bone loss, and not precise single measurements, that is important in determining the treatment regimen.

MANAGEMENT

The best approach for managing osteoporosis and osteopenia is prevention, and it should be stressed that women in their thirties and forties should already be taking calcium supplements to maintain adequate bone mass. Exercise and stress on the bones are equally important in preventing bone loss. Other components of therapy remain subjects of controversy. However, most clinicians agree that intake of approximately 1200 to 1500 mg of calcium per day, 400 units of vitamin D per day and estrogens will prevent appreciable bone loss and fractures if this regimen is initiated immediately after menopause. These recommendations, however, definitely do not increase bone mass, only preventing appreciable loss. Other recommendations have included the use of sodium fluoride, calcitonin and, most recently, electrical stimulation (7–9). However, an overt increase in bone mass has not been consistently observed with these treatment regimens. It has been claimed that the gluconate salt is the most desirable form of calcium for replacement therapy, followed by calcium carbonate and other calcium salts. An easy way to increase the intake of calcium is to use the antacid Tums, which provides approximately 200 mg of calcium per pill; Tums are certainly less expensive than the other preparations, and they also soothe irritated gastric mucosa.

Orthopedic surgeons are faced with managing the complications of osteopenia and osteoporosis, primarily fractures in the elderly. In most cases, a fracture of a vertebral body can be managed with a short period of bedrest (one to two days) and use of an analgesic, followed by gradual mobilization. A back corset is often helpful in relieving pain initially but should be discarded as soon as the pain has subsided to prevent further, diffuse osteopenia. Many elderly patients have difficulty using standard hyperextension braces because they often cause undue pressure over the sternum. Therefore, when a corset is recommended, the patient should be allowed to try it on and also consider other types of brace that provide the same support. Some braces have shoulder straps that relieve the pressure over the sternum and may be more comfortable and easier to apply. Also, the use of a transcutaneous nerve stimulator with the surface electrodes positioned around the thoracic muscles during the initial phase of pain seems to decrease the need for oral analgesics and often allows for early mobilization. Most patients should be free of pain in approximately four to six weeks. Again, it is important to note that other causes of such fractures, including malignant lesions and infection, must be ruled out before it can be assumed that a fracture is due to osteoporosis.

Other fractures directly related to osteopenia include those of the wrists and hips.

HIP FRACTURES

Approximately 175,000 elderly Americans, primarily women, fracture a hip each year. Although advanced technology in surgical and medical managment has decreased the perioperative mortality of such patients to less than 10 percent there is still an overall 40 to 50 percent one-year mortality. Several factors seem to be related to this high mortality, including advanced age, concomitant health problems and, discovered most recently, a psychosocial component that has an important role in overall survival. Studies done in Europe (10,11) have demonstrated that the ability of a patient to shop and have a family member or friend live at the patient's home after the operation is a more important predictor of long-term survival than are strictly "medical" considerations. In a study of patients age 90 or older who had suffered hip fractures, the ability to return home was the single most important factor in promoting long-term survival. One-year survival of those patients did not differ from that of patients between 65 and 90 years of age.

Some patients develop a severe phobia of falling after sustaining a fracture, often leading to complete immobility and death within six months following the event. The mechanism of this phobia and the type of patient who is likely to develop it remain obscure. Few studies have been performed to determine what psychosocial variables play a part in overall survival after a hip fracture.

Nonetheless, it is imperative that a multidisciplinary team approach be used immediately after admission (*not at the time of discharge*) in an attempt to deal with the medical and psychosocial variables. In Europe and Canada, geriatric orthopedic inpatient units have been designed to obviate placement in long-term care facilities and to enable patients to regain functional independence by the time of discharge. This approach has been successful in returning patients to their own environments and is less expensive than placement in a long-term care facility.

There are also certain technical considerations. In severely osteopenic patients, fixation of the bone is often difficult, sometimes necessitating the use of bone cement to provide satisfactory stability for early mobilization. Again, early mobilization is the most important consideration in treating patients with fractured hips. In patients with a fracture of the neck of the femur, a metal prosthesis is placed to permit early ambulation. With internal fixation of such a fracture, there is a high risk for loss of the blood supply to the head of the femur, which would necessitate reoperation. This possibility is usually dealt with by use of hemiarthroplasty. In some cases, primary total hip replacement, although difficult, provides earlier mobilization than do more traditional surgical approaches. Aggressive surgical intervention should be considered in most cases, again to provide early mobilization and relief of pain and to prevent the problems of prolonged bedrest, including pneumonia, urinary incontinence and thrombophlebitis.

In addition to technical failures, such as failure of the prosthesis or hardware, potential complications include thrombophlebitis, pulmonary embolism and incontinence, both bowel and bladder. In a recent study by Brody, 15 percent of the patients discharged after treatment for fractured hips had bowel incontinence, and a greater proportion experienced urinary incontinence (12). The etiologic basis of these complications remains obscure. However, use of an indwelling catheter should be avoided to prevent urinary-tract infection. Although this approach may necessitate extra nursing care, there is a high incidence of shock and sepsis after indwelling catheterization.

Some physicians have recently advocated nonoperative treatment of patients who have fractured hips and severe organic brain syndrome, noting that morbidity and mortality are significantly lower with this approach compared to surgical intervention. However, the medical management of hip fractures is extremely labor intensive, necessitating constant care to prevent formation of decubitus ulcers and other complications of prolonged bedrest. This form of management should be used only in the few facilities that have this capability. In most cases, surgical management affords rapid relief of pain, allows early mobilization and involves less care than does medical management.

In summary, an elderly patient who has a fractured hip should be treated aggressively, not only by the surgeon and physician but by all other members of a multidisciplinary team. This approach prevents some of the psychosocial problems that may have a strong influence on the outcome of such patients.

Hip disease in elderly patients can be severely, debilitating, limiting ambulation and participation in the activities of daily living. With improvements in surgical technique, this dependence can be minimized. The risks of surgical management far outweigh the risks for loss of function and independence.

REFERENCES

1. Harris, W.H., Salzman, E.W., and DeSanctis, R.W. The prevention of thromboembolic disease by prophylactic anticoagulation; a controlled study in elective hip surgery. *J. Bone Joint Surg.* 49A:81–91, 1967.
2. DeLee, S.C. and Rockwood, C.A. Current concepts review; the rise of asprin in thromboembolic disease. *J. Bone Joint Surg.* 62A:149–153, 1980.
3. Evarts, C.M. *Thromboembolic disease.* Vol 28 of American Academy of Orthopedic Surgeons instructional course lectures. St. Louis, C.V. Mosby, 1979, pp. 67–71.
4. Goldhaber, S.Z. *Pulmonary embolism and deep venous thrombosis.* Philadelphia, W.B. Saunders, 1985, pp. 135–138.
5. Vinazzer, H., Loew, D., Simma, W., and Brucke, D. Prophylaxis of postoperative thromboembolism by low dose heparin and by acetylsalicylic acid given simultaneously; a double blind study. *Thromb. Res.* 17:177–184, 1980.
6. Leyvraz, P.F., Richard, J., Bachmann, F., Van Melle, G., Treyvand, J.M., Livio, J.J. and Candardjis, G. Adjusted versus fixed dose subcutaneous heparin in the prevention of deep vein thrombosis after total hip replacement. *N. Engl. J. Med.* 309:954–961, 1983.
7. Brighton, C. The use of electrical stimulation in the treatment of osteoporosis.'' Presented at Them Ol' Bones II; A National Multidisciplinary Conference on Musculoskeletal Diseases in the Aged, Phoenix, 1985.
8. Adams, G.M., and DeVries, H.A. Physiological effects of an exercise training regimen upon women aged 52 to 79. *J. Gerontol.* 28:50–55, 1973.
9. Avioli, L. *The Osteoporotic Syndrome: Detection, Prevention, Treatment.* New York, Grune Publications, 1983.
10. Ceder, L., Thorngren, K.G. Wallden, B. Prognostic indicators and early home rehabilitation in elderly patients with hip fractures. *Clin. Orthop.* 152:173–184.
11. Nickens, H. A review of factors affecting occurrence and outcome of hip fracture with special reference to psychosocial issues. *J. Amer. Geriatr. Soc.* 31:166–170, 1983.
12. Brody, S.J. Post-operative outcome in patients with a fractured hip. Presented at Them Ol' Bones III, Phoenix, 1986.

Chapter 6

John Baum

Knee

PHYSICAL FINDINGS

The knees, being the largest joints in the body, are affected by a great number of metabolic, degenerative and inflammatory disorders. They are involved in most generalized arthritic conditions. In monarticular disease, a knee is most often the affected joint. Because the knees bear a large proportion of body weight, they also are often involved in trauma. As a corollary, if the knees are affected by an arthritic condition, ambulation is inhibited, creating an impact on the activities of daily living. In this situation the usual medical therapy must be extended to incorporate measures to protect and strengthen the joints and associated muscles so that function can be maintained as much as possible.

Diseases of the knees can be divided into those of inflammatory and those of mechanical origin. However, the latter category may include conditions that interfere with function, such as degenerative joint disease, a condition that may have an inflammatory component.

Knee involvement can be monarticular, or it may be a component of polyarticular disease. The discussion in this chapter will first concentrate on monarticular disease and then consider generalized disease in which knee involvement occurs. Finally, rare conditions will be discussed.

As with all types of arthritis, the cardinal signs and symptoms of inflammation in the knees are swelling, warmth, redness, pain and loss of function. It should be noted that knee pain may be the first symptom of ipsilateral hip disease. A careful examination of the hip should always be included in an evaluation of a knee problem.

Swelling may be barely perceptible or may be manifested by a gross abnormality. When a knee is massively swollen, the patient occasionally relates inability to bend the joint. If pain is not the major complaint, that will be the case.

When a knee is examined for swelling, one looks for fullness in the suprapatellar area, in the infrapatellar areas below and laterally and in the usual hollow medially and below the level of the patella. If the hand is placed firmly on the suprapatellar pouch and the index finger and thumb are placed on opposite sides of the patella, any fluid in the joint is pushed down to and held below the patella. A quick thrust on top of the patella with the thumb and index finger of the other hand produces a palpable click. This sensation indicates that there was enough fluid to float the patella, so that the thrust makes it hit against the femur. Even if the patella does not float, there still might be between 2 and 10 ml of fluid present, which can be detected by the "bulge sign." This sign can be elicited in two ways. One method is to "milk" the joint upward two or three times so that fluid is pushed into the suprapatellar pouch. One hand is held medially at the upper border of the patella, while the other hand pushes in and downward against the pouch. If there is any fluid, it is pushed medially and a bulge is seen in the medial hollow below the patella. The other method is to push against the medial side of the joint with the palm and then quickly push laterally with the whole hand. Again, if there is any fluid, a bulge is observed in the medial hollow.

Swelling can be documented by measuring the joint circumference. Measurements of the knee 1 cm above the patella are more easily reproduced than are measurements obtained over the midportion of the patella. The precision of such measurements can be improved by using the mean value of duplicate measurements and by having the same examiner measure the joint each time (1).

Swelling is not always a manifestation of a fluid collection. The author has seen a swollen joint in which fluid could not be demonstrated by clinical means or even by attempting aspiration. In some such cases, the swelling is mostly due to accumulation of synovial tissue.

Abnormally high joint temperature can be determined by comparison to the temperature of the contralateral knee if it appears normal or by comparison to the temperature of the ipsilateral thigh and calf. A novel method for measuring joint temperature is the use of thermography, which must be performed in a room of constant temperature. Before this procedure can be performed, the patient must stay in the room for some time to allow body temperature to equilibrate. For this reason, this technique has been used almost exclusively for research.

Redness can be a useful sign because it is a clue to the diagnosis of several conditions. Redness is infrequently observed in degenerative disease and in conditions of mechanical origin, with the exception of hemiarthrosis, which can produce signs that mimic inflammation. Redness is observed in virtually all inflammatory states but not in all cases of inflammation. Children are more likely than adults to show redness, but even in adults, it is an infrequent finding. Redness seems to develop most often when the inflammation is acute, for example, in rheumatic fever, septic arthritis and gouty arthritis. Gout is accompanied by a purplish red coloration, whereas septic arthritis is evidenced by a bright redness. Swelling and redness of a joint do not necessarily indicate arthritis. The author recently saw a patient undergoing long-term hemodialysis who experienced episodes of joint swelling in the past that were probably related to osteoarthritis, an observation based on the fluid that was aspirated. On presentation, she related that she fell on her knee after undergoing a hemodialysis treatment. The knee became swollen within an hour and had not responded to local application of heat. Physical examination showed diffuse swelling above and over the knee. It was warm, red and tender. Insertion of a needle into the joint seemed to indicate an absence of fluid, but aspiration as the needle was withdrawn produced blood that did not clot. The use of heparin during the hemodialysis treatment evidently had caused a subcutaneous bleed that mimicked joint effusion. Redness is, of course, of dubious diagnostic usefulness in patients with pigmented skin, although if the coloartion is intense, it can be identified.

Pain should be distinguished from tenderness in an examination of a joint. Tenderness is evidenced by applying pressure over the joint. In cases of synovitis, tenderness is demonstrated by applying pressure to the suprapatellar area. Tenderness over the joint margins may be encountered in degenerative joint disease. If tenderness is revealed by applying pressure over the patella, chondromalacia patellae may be the cause. Pain occurs with forced motion of the patella. This symptom can be determined only objectively, by examining the patient in a recumbent position and moving the knee through the full range of motion.

Loss of function is an important sign because it may be the only objective evidence of disability or the only sign that can be monitored to follow up the response to therapy. It is essential that a goniometer be used to determine the angles of maximal flexion and extension. A long-armed instrument must be employed because the reference points for using the goniometer, the greater trochanter and the malleolus, are distant from the knee joint. An alternative method for measuring the angle of maximal flexion is to use a tape measure to determine the distance from the buttock to the heel.

Monarticular disease has changed over the years. In the early part of this century, tuberculosis was a relatively common cause of monarthritis of the knee. It should be pointed out that monarthritis is not exclusively a disease of the knees; theoretically, it can almost any joint. Fletcher and Scott found that a knee was involved in 74 percent of 151 cases of monarticular disease (2). The next most frequently affected joints, the wrists and ankles, were involved in only about 8 percent of cases each. These investigators found that the largest group of cases were due to synovitis of unknown origin. Almost the same proportion of cases (29 percent) were due to "osteoarthrosis," the British term for degenerative joint disease. The third most frequent cause was rheumatoid arthritis (9 percent of cases). This study was done with adult patients. If children were studied, the most frequent cause of monarthritis of the knee would be found to be trauma. Septic arthritis is probably the most frequent cause of inflammatory monarthritis of the knee.

TRAUMATIC CONDITIONS OF THE KNEE

Traumatic conditions in the area of the knees in elderly patients can be divided into those of bony and those of soft-tissue origin. The most common bony injuries are fractures, particularly of the distal condyles of the femur and tibial plateau. Distal fractures of the femur may be missed, particularly when they are superimposed on other fractures of the same leg, especially around the proximal aspect of the bone. This observation is of particular importance in patients with severe dementia, who are unable to give an adequate history, and in those in whom physical examination is extremely difficult because of lack of cooperation or severe joint contractures. Pain and swelling are prominent findings that are often associated with hemarthrosis. A simple way to detect an intra-articular fracture of any joint is to aspirate the hemarthrosis. An aspirate that shows fat globules floating on top of blood is pathognomonic of an intra-articular fracture.

The primary goal of management for most intra-articular fractures, particularly those in elderly patients, is rigid stabilization of the fracture, followed by early immobilization of the limb and early range of motion of the involved joint. Recent reports have stated that continuous passive motion is extremely helpful in obtaining early range of motion. Continuous passive motion is also helpful in nourishing the healing articular cartilage and promotes healing of the articular surface.

Fractures of the patella and of the plateau of the tibia are managed in a similar fashion. In occasional cases, a fracture of the patella is too comminuted to be fixed internally, necessitating partial or complete patellectomy to allow early range of motion of the joint.

Ligamentous injuries and internal derangements of the knees are most frequently encountered in young athletes but are also seen in elderly patients. A typical patient is an elderly man with long-standing degenerative disease of a knee who presents with an abrupt onset of increasing pain and swelling of the joint. In most such cases, there is a history of minimal trauma, such as twisting or turning.

Physical examination demonstrates mild effusion and findings associated with degenerative joint disease as well as extreme tenderness along the medial joint line, particularly on rotation of the tibia. McMurray's test may be positive.

The most common finding on arthroscopic examination is an acute tear of a degenerated medial meniscus, most commonly located in the posterior or posteromedial horn. Removal of the torn meniscus does not affect the course of the disease but can alleviate mechanical stress and symptoms. Arthroscopy has also been useful in the management of other diseases of the knees, including osteoarthritis, rheumatoid arthritis, loose bodies and, occasionally, infection. In most elderly patients undergoing arthroscopic examination, a tourniquet is *not* used in an effort to help prevent deep-vein thrombosis. Although arthroscopy relieves pain in patients with arthritis of the knee, the mechanism of this beneficial result remains obscure. Some investigators believe that the removal of loose debris decreases the inflammatory response, whereas others claim that the vigorous lavage that takes place during the procedure relieves pain by producing denervation of the joint lining.

OSTEONECROSIS

Another disease of the knees that should be considered in elderly patients is osteonecrosis of either the femoral condyle or tibial plateau. The symptoms of this condition similar to those of arthritis and include an aching pain with weight bearing and occasional loss of motion. However, physical examination does not reveal any of the usual findings seen in arthritic conditions. The most common findings are mild effusion with marked tenderness on palpation of the medial condyle or the medial aspect of the plateau. This tenderness is frequently confused with jointline tenderness, often leading to an incorrect diagnosis of a torn meniscus.

Radiographs are frequently normal on initial evaluation. In later stages, there may be flattening of the weight-bearing surface of the medial condyle of the femur, often accompanied by subchondral sclerosis (Figure 6.1). In severe cases, there may be marked arthritis of the medial compartment. The osteochondrosis often seen in young patients is infrequently encountered in the elderly.

A definitive diagnosis can be made by using a labeled bone scan, which consistently demonstrates a "hot area" in the involved bone. Management involves partial or complete restriction of weight bearing for six to eight weeks with the involved joint placed in a knee immobilizer. In most cases, radiographic progression is not noted and the lesion heals. However, some cases show further deterioration at the medial compartment. In such cases, surgical correction by means of tibial or unicompartmental knee replacement may be necessary. Drilling of the osteochondral fragment, occasionally with use of a bone graft, a procedure used in adolescents, does not appear to be helpful in elderly patients. Although the etiologic basis of this condition remains obscure, a likely possibility is recurrent microtrauma leading to the development of a microfracture and vascular compromise to the involved condyle or tibial plateau.

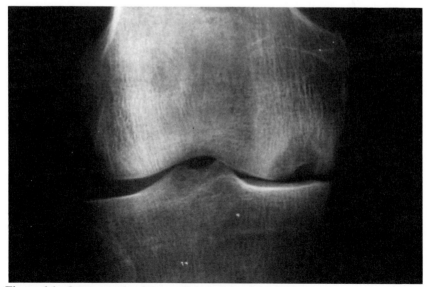

Figure 6.1. Osteonecrosis of the medial condyle of the femur.

Surgical options for the management of osteoarthritis and other forms of arthritis of the knees in elderly patients include arthroscopy, debridement of the joint and removal of predisposing conditions and mechanical factors (i.e., torn meniscus) in moderate cases or proximal tibial osteotomy or unicompartmental or tricompartmental joint replacement in severe cases. The decision to operate is based largely on a patient's degree of pain and level of activity and on the physical and radiographic findings. The choice between osteotomy and joint replacement depends on level of activity. High tibial osteotomy is the preferred surgical treatment in very active patients because loosening of the prosthesis is a major risk after replacement operations. In patients with severe deformities caused by disease in the medial compartment, modification of footwear is of little help.

Approximately 80,000 total knee replacements are now being performed annually in the United States, most of them in elderly patients. Complications are no more common in elderly than in young patients and include thrombotic phenomena, pulmonary embolism and aseptic or septic loosening of the prosthesis. Management of these problems has been mentioned in the chapter on the hips. In about 80 to 90 percent of cases, total knee replacement provides relief of pain and increased mobility. Nonetheless, because of the complexity of the knee joint, the results of the operation are not as good as the results of total hip replacement. New prostheses and greater technical skill may provide better results in the future.

DEGENERATIVE JOINT DISEASE

The major knee problem in the elderly is degenerative joint disease. This disease is not always symptomatic, but radiographic studies show evidence of degenerative changes in a large proportion of the elderly population (Figure 6.2). Nonetheless, all too often complaints centered around a knee prompt the examiner to order radiographs, which are then used as the basis for the diagnosis. For this reason, a number of points deserve emphasis at this juncture. Degenerative joint disease is encountered primarily, but not exclusively, in elderly women.

In the elderly some degree of degenerative joint disease is almost universal. This does not necessarily mean they have symptoms, but whether or not they do, X-ray films will show evidence of degenerative changes. Unfortunately the diagnosis of DJD is made all too often with any complaints in the region of the knee. A routine film is used as the basis for the diagnosis. However there are a number of points in the history and physical examination that should be emphasized. DJD is a disease of older females and is less frequently found in elderly males. Besides gender, obesity is also an important factor. It probably has its effect in females by increasing the stress on a joint that already has about 15 degrees of angulation. This is a result of the wider pelvis in females so that the basic habitus is knock-knees. The frequency is higher in males who have a history of trauma. This can be due to a specific insult such as an

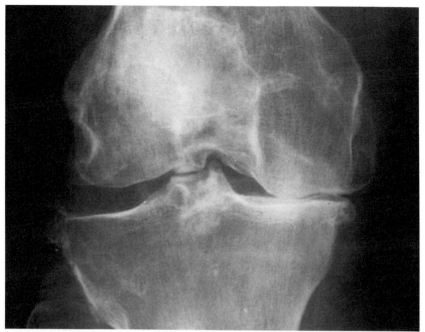

Figure 6.2. Degenerative joint disease of the knee. There is loss of the joint space in the lateral compartment and marked formation of osteophytes.

accident but can also be related to occupational stress. Obesity predisposes to the development of this disease, probably leading to a much higher proportion of cases in women by increasing the stress on joints that already have about 15 degrees of angulation. Men with a history of trauma, either a specific insult, such as an accident, or an event relating to occupational stress, are at relatively increased risk for the development of the disease.

In recent years, there has been debate regarding the increased stress placed on the knees because of the preoccupation with fitness, especially jogging. However Fries and colleagues and other investigators (3) have found that such activity does not lead to symptomatic disease. Those authors found only a slight increase in the density of the joint ends of the femur and the tibia and a slight increase in osteophyte formation but, most importantly, observed no decrease in the joint space. The latter finding indicates that there is no excessive wear of the cartilage. Nonetheless, prolonged, vigorous running can increase the risk for certain injuries, for example hairline fractures, and damage to soft-tissue structures, such as ligaments and tendons.

A number of primary conditions can lead to secondary osteoarthritis of the knees (Table 6.1).

Among the metabolic disorders, hemochromatosis may be encountered most frequently but because all these conditions are rare, statistics are of little diagnostic

TABLE 6.1 Causes of Secondary
Osteoarthritis of the Knees

Heritable metabolic disorders
Wilson's disease
Hemochromatosis
Morquio's syndrome
Multiple epiphyseal dysplasia
Neuropathic arthropathy (Charcot's joints)
Hemophilic arthropathy
Acromegalic arthropathy
Paget's disease (osteitis deformans)
Rheumatoid arthritis
Gout
Septic and tuberculous arthritis
Trauma

utility. The author has seen cases of these metabolic disorders but feels that hemochromatosis is likely to present as osteoarthritis before the primary condition is diagnosed. Radiographs often demonstrate chondrocalcinosis, but this finding is not diagnostic. It has been claimed that at least half of patients with hemochromatosis also show chondrocalcinosis. The author has seen a patient with a hip prosthesis in whom hemochromatosis was not diagnosed until he returned for an operation on the other hip. A review of the tissue from the initial operation revealed the typical large deposits of iron in the synovial tissue.

Neuropathic arthropathy, better known as Charcot's joint, is due to a loss of proprioceptive and pain fibers. Some patients retain the sensation of pain. Although Charcot's joint is historically associated with tabes dorsalis, this degenerative disease is no longer a major cause. Charcot's joint is encountered in diabetics with peripheral neuropathy, but it usually involves the foot and ankle in this disease. The most frequent cause of this condition today is syringomyelia, although the latter disease is more likely to involve the arms. By contrast, congenital indifference to pain, paraplegia and Charcot-Marie-Tooth disease are most likely to involve the legs.

These conditions start with swelling and deformity of the joints. Acute episodes can occur. Physical examination reveals what has been referred to as a "bag of bones," or loose bodies within the affected joints. There is substantial formation of new bone with a major deformity of the joints. Surgical management is difficult but occasionally helps.

Hemophilic arthropathy mainly affects young persons, but in long-standing cases in adults, the cartilage becomes damaged because of blood in the joints. There is also bleeding into surrounding structures. Progression of the arthropathy leads not only to degenerative joint disease but also, on occasion, to ankylosis and osteoporosis. In elderly patients, the extensive joint damage is major evidence of past acute episodes.

Acromegaly results in incongruity of the joints and, in turn, changes typical of osteoarthritis. One must always be careful when making what appears to be an obvious diagnosis. The author once saw an elderly patient with easily recognizable acromegaly. She had effusion in both knees. A rheumatologist eager to teach the residents the importance of clinical observation noted that a patient with obvious acromegaly must also have degenerative joint disease. Aspiration yielded inflammatory joint fluid of low viscosity that had a high white cell count. The correct diagnosis was confirmed by laboratory tests, which showed rheumatoid factor and an elevated erythrocyte sedimentation rate.

Although incongruity of the joints is an obvious direct cause leading to osteoarthritis, another, indirect cause of osteoarthritis is Paget's disease, which strikes the long bones in the legs, leading to secondary changes in the joints. The result can be knock-knees or bowlegs, and the distortion in the joints leads to degenerative changes.

RHEUMATOID ARTHRITIS

Rheumatoid arthritis is a systemic disease that can involve all the joints. Although it characteristically is evidenced by all the signs and symptoms of inflammation (i.e., swelling, warmth, redness, pain and loss of function), these manifestations may not be noticeable in elderly patients.

In elderly patients, the disease may have started anytime, even during childhood as juvenile arthritis. However, in most cases, the disease has started in adulthood. Rheumatoid arthritis is less common in men than in women, in whom it usually starts during the childbearing years. The status of an elderly patient who has had rheumatoid arthritis since relatively early in life depends on the course the disease has taken.

One form of the disease begins suddenly, is severe and appears to become quiescent within one or two years. Restriction of motion may be a permanent consequence, and there is residual thickening of the structures around the joints in occasional cases. In this form, the course can resemble that of degenerative joint disease because the joint damage has the same secondary effect.

In the episodic form, periods of disease activity alternate with periods of remission. Although secondary degeneration can develop in old age, there are enough recurrences of active inflammation to make control of the rheumatoid arthritis the major concern to patients with this form. The knees may be bulky, suggesting osteoarthritis, but they are warm, tender and painful with motion, and the joints contain inflammatory synovial fluid.

If more precise identification of the disease process is desired, joint aspiration is necessary. The characteristics of the fluid define the form of the disease.

In rheumatoid arthritis, the fluid is so cloudy that it is almost impossible to see through the tube. This cloudiness is the result of cells and various tissue breakdown products in the fluid. The next step is to determine the viscosity of the fluid. In cases of inflammation, the viscosity is poor, as demonstrated by rubbing one or two drops between the thumb and index finger. If the fluid feels thin, its poor viscosity can be confirmed by separating the digits. Thin fluid produces strings that break before they reach about an inch in length. Normal synovial fluid feels thick and sticky and produces longer strings.

Elderly patients usually present during an acute attack, which should be managed with a nonsteroidal anti-inflammatory drug (NSAID). As was noted earlier, such patients should be started on a dosage below what is recommended in the package insert. They may respond favorably to a lower dosage, and there is less chance of side effects at such a dosage.

The author has seen a few patients in whom rheumatoid arthritis has had an unremitting course. By old age, most such patients show severe joint destruction despite what appears to be limited disease activity. An NSAID is occasionally helpful in such cases, but if the knee destruction is marked, surgical intervention probably is required.

An interesting group of patients with swollen knees are those over age 65. Some such patients show the characteristic changes of osteoarthritis. If they have had arthritis, the chief complaints are severe pain, significant restriction of motion and, perhaps, increased warmth. An important question to ask while taking the history is whether there has been any change in morning stiffness. In cases of osteoarthritis, there is typically morning stiffness, but it rarely lasts more than 30 minutes. If the stiffness lasts more than about an hour an inflammatory process has supervened. Rheumatoid arthritis is the most likely candidate, especially if both knees are involved. If the joints contain fluid, the diagnosis is best determined by aspirating the joints, as was noted earlier.

Recently, an excellent study was performed in Boston to determine the clinical features of "elderly-onset rheumatoid arthritis" (4). More than 200 patients in whom the disease began after age 60 (average patient age, 67.2) were compared with a group in whom the disease began before age 59 (average patient age, 46.6).

Characteristics of the older patient group included abrupt onset (twice as sudden as in the younger patient group), a higher incidence of involvement of the large joints, a higher incidence of a greater initial elevation of the erythrocyte sedimentation rate and a lower incidence of rheumatoid factor. Treatment was similar in both groups. However, according to the authors, the most interesting finding was that "the outcome of the elderly-onset group assessed at the last visit was significantly better than that of the younger-onset group across a variety of pertinent disease outcome measures." This important finding indicates that physicians have reason to encourage their patients and should treat them vigorously. It may be that when rheumatoid arthritis starts in old age, it tends to begin suddenly and rapidly go into remission. The authors believe that such cases may represent a distinct form of the disease in elderly patients. Another possibility is that such cases do not represent true rheumatoid arthritis but, instead, either a form of polymyalgia rheumatica characterized by prominent joint rather than muscle complaints or palindromic rheumatism. The latter condition is a form of episodic arthritis in which the joint signs and symptoms are of short duration. About half of patients with this condition later suffer from persistent rheumatoid arthritis. However, in a report from London, only two of 39 patients were over age 60, and knee involvement was not observed in either patient (5).

In polyarticular presentations of rheumatoid arthritis in elderly patients, involvement of the knees is seen in 52 percent of cases, an incidence exceeded only by that of the metacarpophalangeal joints and wrists (6).

There are other interesting observations. Cases of short duration (i.e., one year or less) involve the shoulders, elbows, wrists and knees much more frequently between ages 65 and 75 than other ages. Only in this age range are the knees affected; the small joints are also involved at other ages (7). This pattern of involvement also was most likely to evolve to mild disease in old age.

Treatment of elderly patients depends on whether the knees are involved and must take into account a number of considerations. In unusual cases in which only one joint is involved, aspiration to confirm the diagnosis, followed by intra-articular instillation of a long-acting corticosteroid is probably advisable. In cases of active synovitis, this approach constitutes only symptomatic therapy, which reduces effusion, relieves pain and allows participation in active physical therapy. Intra-articular administration of a corticosteroid is also helpful if only a few large joints show disease activity, particularly if severe involvement of one or both knees interferes with a patient's activity or therapy.

In a study at Oxford, hydrocortisone was injected into the knees of patients with rheumatoid synovitis, and the range of motion of the joints was carefully measured (8). The use of this agent, which is not a long-acting preparation, increased the range of flexion during walking, a change that persisted appreciably for eight weeks. Pain was relieved before the maximal effect on joint function had been achieved. In this study, a control group received saline in place of the corticosteroid. There was a significant difference between the responses of the two patient groups. Thus, instillation of a corticosteroid is more effective than aspiration alone.

All recently introduced corticosteroids have a longer period of action than does hydrocortisone. Three of the newer agents, prednisone *t*-butyl acetate, methylprednisone acetate and triamcinolone hexacetonide, have been tested by a group in Bath, England (9). The responses to these three drugs were similar, except for minor differences in overall improvement and relief of morning stiffness, during a two-week trial. Thermographic studies, which may be helpful in determining the severity of inflammation, showed much greater improvement with triamcinolone, and this drug was effective up to 28 days. In addition, the noninjected, contralateral knee displayed improvement. It must be assumed the improvement in the noninjected knee was due to absorption of the drug. Moreover, triamcinolone had the least effect of the three agents on endogenous plasma levels of cortisol at one month. The authors thus concluded that triamcinolone has definite advantages over the two other drugs.

The typical patient with rheumatoid arthritis has polyarticular involvement.

Thus in most cases of the disease, management is more complex. Initial therapy consists of an NSAID and physical therapy. To this regimen is then added a long-acting drug, such as *d*-penicillamine, hydroxychloroquine, a gold compound, azathioprine or, the newest one, methotrexate. Use of these agents reduces inflammation and inhibits involvement of additional joints, but their effectiveness on a specific joint, such as a knee, is not predictable. Therefore, even when a long-acting drug is used, therapy should be directed at individual joints. As was noted previously, adjuvant therapy includes intra-articular injection of the joint with a corticosteroid. This approach should be used, however, only if there is a specific problem, such as difficulty walking. Therapy should be individualized to take into consideration the needs of a given patient. A woman with young children or a working person would be proper candidates for such an approach. A note of caution, however: a joint should not be injected more often than every three months. More frequent instillation of a corticosteroid may lead to the development of Charcot's joint, probably because overusage of such agents almost eliminates all pain and promotes degeneration of cartilage. Although the initial response to long-acting corticosteroids may last several months, with each successive injection, the duration of action progressively shortens until the beneficial effect lasts only a few weeks. At this point, or preferably before it is reached, the patient should be followed up by an orthopedist for consideration as a surgical candidate for synovectomy.

Physical therapy is an important part of the management of any form of arthritis of the knees, be it an inflammatory variant, such as rheumatoid arthritis, or one that restricts motion almost solely because of pain, such as osteoarthritis. It is difficult to get elderly patients to participate in an active treatment program because many of them are relatively inactive, in some cases as a result of the restriction posed by the disease.

The author recommends to such patients a simple isometric exercise program for the quadriceps muscle. While they are watching television, they are instructed to extend both legs alternately or simultaneously when a commercial message appears. They hold up their legs throughout the message and lower them slowly when it ends. Alternatively, one leg may be raised at a time. This exercise is a simple one, but to assure compliance, it helps to have someone in the household provide encouragement. More complicated exercise programs that require the use of weights are best done under the supervision of a physical therapist. Patients are taught that even with arthritis, they will be able to do more with stronger muscles.

External supports, such as Ace bandages and knee braces, are not helpful unless there is severe joint instability. The use of braces promotes further muscle atrophy and deterioration of the joint. Some braces even severely constrict the area around the joint, causing edema and increasing the risk for thromboembolic phenomena. Therefore, supports should be used only in conjunction with vigorous physical activity or in cases in which the knee demonstrates severe laxity.

Even though gout is listed in Table 6.1 as a form of secondary osteoarthritis, this condition is best considered as a type of crystal arthritis. Classifying gout in this manner necessitates the inclusion of pseudogout, which is caused mainly by deposition of calcium pyrophosphate crystals. A less common form of crystal arthritis is caused by deposition of calcium apatite crystals.

GOUT AND PSEUDOGOUT

Gout is a well-known disease whose frequency has been declining in recent years. Certainly, the recent awareness of the need to reduce intake of total calories and protein has resulted in a decrease in the levels of purines, thus slowing the accumulation of their metabolic end product, uric acid. However, such altered dietary habits may only delay the accumulation of uric acid until old age, possibly leading to a higher frequency of gouty attacks in elderly persons.

Of 1077 patients with gout in one study, 20.6 percent of the men (about 85 percent of all patients) had the onset at age 65 or older (10). Among women in the study, the disease began at or after age 65 in 45.2 percent of cases! In some cases, the gout was secondary to a chronic blood disorder that is accompanied by a high turnover of purines, such as chronic leukemia or polycythemia. About 10 percent of the patients were thought to have secondary gout. In 7 percent of 600 of the patients, the first attack occurred in a knee, and this joint was involved in an attack 19.9 percent of the time. Therefore, the knees are ultimately involved in patients with gout.

Gout can be diagnosed on the basis of the history, especially if family members have had the disease or if a commonly affected joint, such as that of the great toe, is involved. The finding of tophi is a pathognomonic sign. Radiographs show typical changes when the disease is well established. Although the use of colchicine is a time-honored management approach, it can cause unique problems in elderly patients. The side effect of diarrhea may be devastating in such patients. Although it may be useful in a therapeutic trial, as in the previously cited study, the drug failed to give the classic rapid response in about one-thrid of patients. In an acute attack, it is preferable to try to obtain fluid, which can be examined for intracellular uric acid crystals to obtain a definitive diagnosis. Synovial fluid can be kept in the cold for several hours before examination. Most NSAIDS (with the exception of salicylates) are effective in managing attacks of gouty arthritis.

Long-term therapy involves the use of an uricosuric agent or a xanthine oxidase inhibitor. The widespread use of drugs to manage hyperuricemia found on routine blood tests may help explain the decreased incidence of gout in recent years. Some hematologists believe that it is advisable to lower the blood level of uric acid in patients with myeloproliferative diseases. However, many rheumatologists believe that only excessively high blood levels of uric acid warrant management. Even if the blood level is merely above normal, the disease may not develop. The use of such drugs can provoke side effects, although their incidence is low.

Pseudogout, which is caused by deposition of calcium pyrophosphate crystals in joints, is truly a disease of the elderly. Deposition of this material in the joint cartilage is known as chondrocalcinosis. In a study of 76 women and 29 men with this disease, the mean age was 73 among the women and 62 among the men (11). Only 18 patients were younger than 60 years of age.

In most reported series, there is radiographic evidence of chondrocalcinosis, manifested by a thin, stippled band on the cartilage surface (Figure 6.3).

Among patients with pseudogout, there is also a high incidence of other diseases and precipitating factors. However, it seems that many associated conditions may be coincidental findings. There have been reports that attacks are provoked by trauma, infection and surgical intervention. However, pseudogout is undoubtedly associated with some diseases because of the high frequency of both conditions together. For example, about 25 percent of patients with hyperparathyroidism show evidence of chondrocalcinosis on radiographic examination. Elderly patients are most likely to show these conditions in combination. As was noted earlier, about half of patients with hemochromatosis and arthritis also have chondrocalcinosis.

Pseudogout can present in different ways. The term refers to acute gouty attacks in patients with calcium pyrophosphate crystals. A small proportion of patients with pseudogout show polyarticular involvement and signs and symptoms of inflammation that resemble those of rheumatoid arthritis. For example, they have prolonged morning stiffness and may even show erosion of the joint, making the diagnosis difficult. Serologic studies may compound the confusion because such studies can demonstrate a low titer of rheumatoid factor and elevation of the erythrocyte sedimentation rate in many elderly patients. In the

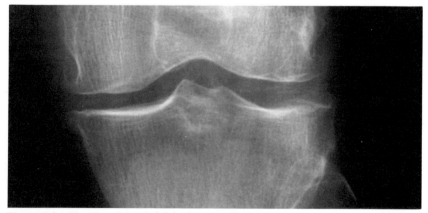

Figure 6.3. Chondrocalcinosis of the knee cartilage.

largest group of patients, degenerative joint disease develops later. Because the knees show the most severe involvement in primary cases of this disease, these joints also show the greatest involvement in the secondary form. Just as a radiograph that shows osteophytes is not necessarily evidence of symptomatic disease, radiographic evidence of chondrocalcinosis does not necessarily result in symptomatic disease. In both situations, however, clinical manifestations can develop later.

Management is accomplished with an NSAID. Because pseudogout is a crystal-induced form of arthritis, there have been attempts to manage it with colchicine, but the results have been poor. Some authors have claimed that the disease can be managed with colchicine given intravenously, but this method of administration requires care. Aspiration of an acutely inflamed joint is both a diagnostic and a therapeutic procedure because the fluid so obtained can be analyzed to demonstrate crystals and removal of the fluid eliminates the acute gouty attacks. Thus, it is advisable to remove as much fluid as possible from an inflamed joint.

The last category is concerned with septic joints. Tuberculous arthritis is now rarely encountered in the United States because the incidence of tuberculosis has decreased dramatically. Extrapulmonary tuberculosis is seen in about 50 percent of patients with joint disease. About 15 percent of such patients show knee involvement, with most of the bone disease being in the spine. The disease begins insidiously with joint pain and a limp; these manifestations are initially intermittent but later become permanent. In most cases, the diagnosis of tuberculosis is already established. For this reason, any joint involvement in such patients is tuberculous until proved otherwise.

The diagnosis requires aspiration of the joint and culture of the aspirate. In the author's experience, a biopsy and culture of the synovial tissue are equally important. The author has seen negative fluid cultures from patients in whom the organism has been identified in not only the tissue but also in cultures of the tissue.

Management involves the adminsitration of an antituberculous drug for as long as three years, especially if there is bone involvement. Immobilization in a cast for eight to 20 weeks has also been recommended along with nonweight-bearing activity. In patients with severe disease accompanied by joint destruction, the joint should be fused.

Septic arthritis is a threat in debilitated elderly patients. It has been pointed out that septic arthritis in elderly patients is usually associated with some other joint disease that destroys the normal joint architecture or with a disease that reduces the normal defense mechanisms, such as diabetes (12).

There is a relatively high frequency of joint sepsis due to β-hemolytic streptococci in elderly patients, although sepsis due to staphylococci is reported most often. The infection is usually blood borne, so that the sudden appearance of a hot, swollen, tender joint in a patient with sepsis should arouse suspicion of septic arthritis. Because a joint can be quickly destroyed by infection, joints that show such signs and symptoms should be aspirated, the specimen Gram-stained and the fluid sent for culture; a blood culture should be obtained at the same time. The author has seen cases in which the organism was identified only in the blood culture. An antibiotic to manage infection by the likely culprit should be started. However, the drug should not be injected directly into the joint because a high concentration of an antibiotic may damage the cartilage. An inflamed joint rapidly accumulates enough of an antibiotic for this purpose.

The diagnostic algorithm in Chapter 1 includes pes anserina bursitis. In the author's experience, this condition is a major problem in elderly patients referred to rheumatic disease clinics by primary-care physicians. This syndrome, which frequently causes knee pain when encountered alone or in combination with other conditions, should be recognized and managed by primary-care physicians more often, especially by physicians whose practices are largely geriatric patients. Therapy is simple once the condition has been identified.

REFERENCES

1. Kirwan, J.R., Byron, M.A., Winfield, J., Altman, D.G., and Gumpel, J.M. Circumferential measurements in the assessment of synovitis of the knee. *Rheumatol. Rehabil.* 18:78–84, 1979.
2. Fletcher, M.R., and Scott, J.T. Chronic monarticular synovitis: Diagnostic and prognostic features. *Ann. Rheum. Dis.* 34:171–176, 1975.
3. Lane, N.E., Bloch, D.A., Jones, H.H., Marshall, W.H., Wood, P.D., and Fries, J.F. Long distance running, bone density, and osteoarthritis. *JAMA* 255:1147–1151, 1986.
4. Deal, C.L., Meenan, R.F., Goldenberg, D.L., Anderson, J.J., Sack, B., Pasten, R.S., and Cohen, A.S. The clinical features of elderly onset rheumatoid arthritis: A comparison with younger onset disease of similar duration. *Arthritis Rheum.* 28:978–984, 1985.
5. Wajed, M.A., Brown, D.L., and Currey, H.L.F. Palindromic rheumatism. *Ann. Rheum. Dis.* 36:56–61, 1977.
6. Brown, J.W., and Sones, D.A. The onset of rheumatoid arthritis in the aged. *J. Amer. Geriatr. Soc.* 15:875–881, 1967.
7. Fleming, A., Benn, R.T., Corbett, M., and Wood, P.H.N. Early rheumatoid disease: II. Patterns of joint involvement. *Ann. Rheum Dis.* 35:361–364, 1976.
8. Bossingham, D.H., McQueen, A.K., and Mowat, A.G. Knee function after intra-articular hydrocortisone. *Rheumatol. Rehabil.* 20:90–101, 1981.
9. Bird, H.A., Ring, E.F.J., and Bacon, P.J. A thermographic and clinical comparison of three intra-articular steroid preparations in rheumatoid arthritis. *Ann. Rheum. Dis.* 38:36–39, 1979.
10. Currie, W.J.C. The gout patient in general practice. *Rheumatol. Rehabil.* 17:205–218, 1978.
11. Dieppe, P.A., Jones, H.E., Scott, D.G., Watt, I., Alexander, G.J., Doherty, M., and Manhire, A. Pyrophosphate arthropathy: A clinical and radiological study of 105 cases. *Ann. Rheum. Dis.* 41:371–376, 1982.
12. Sharp, J.T., Lidsky, M.D., Duffy, J., and Duncan, M.W. Infectious arthritis. *Arch. Intern. Med.* 193:1125–1130, 1979.

Chapter 7

Robert R. Karpman

Foot and Ankle

In Chapter 8, it is noted that foot disorders are a common cause of dysmobility in the elderly. Surprisingly enough, elderly people claim that physicians tend to overlook the feet and ankles during physical examinations. The need for a careful and systematic evaluation of the feet and ankles of elderly patients is thus apparent.

The history should include questions relating to gait problems, pain, difficulty with footwear and concurrent medical problems (e.g., diabetes, peripheral vascular disease and arthritis). The physical examination should include an evaluation of gait with and without shoes to determine the cause of any gait disturbances. Shoes should be checked for wear patterns, correct size, stability and comfort. Elderly people on fixed incomes often defer the purchase of proper shoes and often wear shoes having improper sizes, widths or surfaces. In nursing homes, slippers, the most common type of footwear, provide little support for the feet and often contribute to falls on slippery surfaces.

The skin of the feet and ankles should be checked for corns and calluses, ulcers, nail deformities and other abnormalities. Palpation of the peripheral pulses should be a regular part of the examination. Doppler sonography may be necessary for determining the adequacy of blood flow to the feet.

Blood pressure determined in a serial manner from the thighs to the feet in patients suspected of having peripheral vascular disease helps ascertain the ischemic index (1–3). The ischemic index is calculated by dividing the brachial systolic pressure by the pressures in the calf and ankle. If the index is 0.5 or greater, or pressure at the ankle is more than 50 mm Hg, there is a high probability that a wound will heal.

A thorough neurologic examination should be performed to rule out local or generalized impairment. Neurologic problems and their management will be discussed later.

Motor strength of the ankle (dorsiflexion and plantar flexion) and motion of the subtalar joints (inversion and eversion), midfoot and forefoot should be evaluated. The standard range of motion of an ankle is 60 degrees and subtalar motion 50 degrees. Determining the range of motion of the metatarsophalangeal joints, particularly those of the great toes, are important in the diagnosis of hallux rigidus and other arthritic conditions. Deformities, such as hallux valgus, bunions, hammertoes, flat feet and high arched feet, should be noted and the mobility of the toes determined.

When the examination has been completed, a correct diagnosis can be made. In our discussion of the various disorders, a regional approach to the feet and ankles will be used. The regions considered are the ankle, hindfoot, midfoot and forefoot.

THE ANKLE

Apart from traumatic arthritis, noninflammatory arthritides (e.g., degenerative joint disease and osteoarthritis) are rarely found in the ankles, although they are not infrequently seen in other joints of the legs. Therefore, pain and decreased range of motion of an ankle in a patient with no history of trauma suggests an inflammatory disorder.

In rheumatoid arthritis, synovial thickening, swelling, pain and stiffness (usually symmetric) are observed. If there is effusion, the examiner should perform aspiration to rule out deposition diseases, such as chondrocalcinosis and gout, although gout in the ankles is a rare finding. Septic arthritides can develop, particularly in an immunocompromised host, as well as with a chronic granulomatous infection, such as tuberculosis or coccidiodomycosis. These conditions, too, are relatively rare. Other inflammatory arthritides with ankle manifestations (e.g., Reiter's disease and ankylosing spondylitis) are also seen infrequently.

Management of a local disease depends on the underlying disorder. In cases of rheumatoid arthritis with recurrent synovitis and pain, intra-articular administration of a corticosteroid may be helpful. If repeat injections (no closer than three to six months apart) are unsuccessful, synovectomy may be performed. This procedure has recently been done with the aid of an arthroscope; this approach reduces postoperative morbidity and allows for early improvement in range of motion. In cases with complete loss of the joint space, severe pain and limitation of motion, total ankle replacement has been advocated, primarily in patients with rheumatoid arthritis. Total ankle replacement is certainly not as successful as total hip or knee replacement because there is a high incidence of loosening of the prosthesis and loss of motion when the ankle joint is replaced. If subtalar arthritis is severe, total ankle replacement should be considered in place of pantalar fusion to provide at least some range of motion. In severe cases of traumatic arthritis, ankle fusion remains the treatment of choice. Little disability is noted with a solid ankle fusion if the patient is provided with modified footwear that incorporates a rocker-bottom sole or soft ankle cushion heel heel. The ideal placement of the ankle is in the neutral position, both in the antero-posterior and in the lateral plane. However, some women prefer 5 or 10 degrees of plantar flexion to allow for use of low- or mid-heel shoes.

Other common conditions that involve the hindfoot are Achilles tendinitis, rupture of a tendon, retrocalcaneal bursitis and calcaneal spurs. Achilles tendinitis is easy to diagnose; if pain is elicited on palpation of the tendon and there is increased pain on passive extension of the ankle, Achilles tendinitis is the cause. Palpation often reveals thickening of the tendon sheath as well. Management consists of application of ice in acute cases, a heel lift and oral administration of an anti-inflammatory drug. The use of corticosteroids is contraindicated in Achilles tendinitis because there is a high incidence of rupture after intratendinous injection. Should conservative management fail, exploration of the tendon and release of the tendon sheath may be necessary. Rupture of the tendon occurs more often in middle-aged than in elderly patients; however, active elderly patients may rupture the tendon, usually at the musculotendinous junction. The diagnosis relies on palpation of a defect in the tendinous structure, weak plantar flexion and a positive response on Thompson's test, in which the examiner squeezes the gastrocnemius muscle to produce plantar flexion of the foot. If this response does not occur, a rupture should be considered.

The choice between operative and nonoperative management depends on the severity of a rupture and the patient's level of activity. Results are satisfactory with either approach.

Retrocalcaneal bursitis may be confused with Achilles tendinitis; however, in the former condition, pain is usually limited to the area of attachment of the Achilles tendon to the calcaneus. Swelling and redness are frequently observed, and calcium deposits may be seen on roentgenographic studies. Management is essentially the same as for Achilles tendinitis; however, a corticosteroid can be injected into the retrocalcaneal bursa, not the tendon sheath, in refractory cases. Exploration and removal of the bursa are occasionally necessary.

The term heel spur has been used to describe a variety of entities. Asymptomatic spurs on the plantar surface of the calcaneus are visualized by roentgenography in a large proportion of elderly patients. Patients with inflammatory arthritis, such as ankylosing spondylitis or Reiter's syndrome, may have a painful heel spur in addition to other joint complaints. The most common cause of heel pain is plantar fascitis. The plantar fascia originates on the calcaneus and extends along the plantar surface of the foot to attach at the heads of the metatarsal bones and metatarsophalangeal joints. Because the ligaments in the longitudinal arch tend to weaken or stretch after recurrent trauma or, particularly, with advancing age, this fascia tends to become inflamed. In most cases, pain is felt at the attachment of the fascia to the calcaneus. Recurrent stretching or inflammation can produce a traction spur, leading to chronic pain. Most patients with plantar fascitis complain of pain, particularly when rising from bed and taking their first steps. In occasional cases, spasm and cramping of the foot occur.

Plantar fascitis is diagnosed by eliciting pain on palpation of the fascia, particularly at its attachment to the calcaneus, or on passive stretching of the fascia by dorsiflexion of the toes. A spur may be seen on roentgenographic studies. Management consists of oral administration of an anti-inflammatory agent, stretching of the fascia, placement of a horseshoe pad in the shoe to lessen the pressure on the heel and, occasionally, the use of longitudinal arch supports. In approximately 40 to 50 percent of patients, symptoms resolve with such treatment. In recalcitrant cases, injections of a corticosteroid into the origin of the fascia may be beneficial. However, in elderly patients, repeated injections of a corticosteroid should be avoided because such therapy can induce subcutaneous atrophy of the heelpad, leading to serious consequences. In rare instances, removal of the spur and release of the fascia are necessary.

In some cases of medial heel pain, the cause is incorrectly diagnosed as calcaneal spurs when, in fact, the pain is the result of entrapment of the medial calcaneal branch of the posterior tibial nerve. Injection of a local anesthetic into the area may aid in the diagnosis. Surgical release of the entrapped nerve may be necessary.

Loss of the subcutaneous fatpad, leading to recurrent heel pain, frequently occurs in elderly patients. In most cases, this condition can be easily managed with a cushion device, such as Tuli heel cups, or some other type of padding in the shoe.

Calcaneal fractures usually occur in young patients as a result of falling from a height. However, elderly patients with severe osteoporosis may sustain calcaneal fractures as the result of a number of traumatic injuries, for example, in motor vehicle accidents. Management consists of elevation of the involved leg in a plaster splint. Because there are numerous septa in the heelpad, calcaneal fractures can be extremely painful due to formation of a hematoma, and patients may need to be admitted to a hospital for analgesia. Later, a walking cast is used until the fracture has healed, usually in six to eight weeks. Late deformities, particularly valgus deformities of the heel, or subtalar arthritis may occur.

Ankle sprains can be divided into three categories. Grade I sprains consist of mild disruption of a lateral ankle ligament, usually the tibiotalar ligament. Minimal swelling is noted on examination, and management consists of a supportive wrap and progressive ambulation.

Grade III sprains are the most severe and are characterized by complete disruption of the ligaments with instability in the mediolateral and anteroposterior planes secondary to a tear in the anterior joint capsule. Soft-tissue swelling is noted over the medial and lateral aspects of the ankle and foot, and there also is obvious instability. Roentgenograms may demonstrate excessive tilting of the talus on stress views. Management consists of elevation of the leg and application of ice until the swelling has subsided, followed by immobilization in a walking cast for four to six weeks. Open repair has been advocated, particularly in patients who participate in strenuous athletic activity; however, satisfactory results can be obtained with conservative therapy.

Grade II, or second-degree, sprains fall between the two categories just described. In most cases, second-degree sprains should be managed in the same manner as third-degree sprains, with immobilization. This approach usually provides greater comfort and decreases the amount of swelling after the injury, which can otherwise last up to four weeks. A device called an "air cast" has recently been used in place of a plaster or fiberglass cast. This device provides support to the foot and ankle, allows for motion of the ankle and fits into a regular shoe. It is much more comfortable and safe than the traditional devices, particularly in elderly patients. Ace bandages or elastic wraps should not be used in patients with second- or third-degree sprains because they can block venous return, thus increasing swelling, and provide little if any support to the foot or ankle.

Fractures of the ankle in elderly patients are managed in the same way as they are in young patients. Management depends on the mechanism of injury as well as on displacement of the ankle mortise. Internal fixation can often be difficult in cases of severe osteoporosis, and extreme care should be employed. In most cases, however, the joint and leg can be mobilized at an early stage only with open reduction and internal fixation.

THE HINDFOOT

The subtalar joints include the talonavicular, talocalcaneal and calcaneal cuboid joints. These joints are responsible for inversion and eversion of the foot. Arthritis in these joints is generally of traumatic origin or a result of rheumatoid arthritis. Most patients with rheumatoid arthritis of the subtalar joints present with progressive planovalgus, or flatfoot deformity. It becomes difficult to wear shoes, and excessive wear on the medial side of the shoe is noted. In the early stages, management consists of the use of a longitudinal arch support with some type of medial heel wedge. These supports should be placed in an extra-depth shoe with a stiff counter to prevent excessive pronation of the forefoot. A rigid orthosis, such as a rhodur plastic or polypropylene device, is difficult for elderly patients to use; for this reason, an appliance made of cork or a rubber compound should be substituted. In severe cases, fusion of one or more of the subtalar joints is advocated for relief of pain and prevention of further deformity.

Neurologic Disorders

Patients with pain and paresthesias in the ankle fall into one of several groups. Patients with peripheral neuropathy usually have symmetric disease, with the exception of those with diabetes. Appropriate laboratory studies should be performed to define the specific cause of a peripheral neuropathy, for example, diabetes, a thyroid disorder or a vitamin deficiency. Management depends on the underlying cause. In a few instances, phenytoin or pentoxi fylline has been used to relieve the symptoms of peripheral neuropathy. If a diagnosis cannot be made, biopsy of the sural nerve may be necessary.

Radiculopathy that results from herniation of a disk or spinal stenosis can cause paresthesias in the foot and ankle. Reflex changes may be present. The diagnosis and management of radiculopathy have been discussed in a previous chapter.

Vascular insufficiency is another consideration in the differential diagnosis, especially in patients with symptoms of claudication.

Another possibility is compressive neuropathy, particularly of the posterior tibial nerve during its course through the tarsal tunnel. Patients present with pain along the medial side of the foot and ankle radiating into the plantar surface of the foot in the distribution of the medial and lateral plantar nerves. Pain usually occurs after ambulation and frequently is worse at night. Tinel's sign can be elicited on palpation of the medial side of the foot at the level of the tarsal tunnel. The diagnosis may be aided by obtaining nerve conduction velocities and electromyograms. Once the diagnosis has been established, surgical release of the tunnel can help resolve the symptoms, just as relief of symptoms in the hand is aided by release of the carpal tunnel. Paresthesias in the lateral aspect of the foot may be related to compression of the sural nerve, usually a result of scarring from old trauma. Injection of a local anesthetic around the nerve oftens helps in making the diagnosis. Decompression is rarely necessary. Most symptoms usually resolve on administration of an anti-inflammatory agent.

THE MIDFOOT

The midfoot consists of the navicular bone, cuboid bone, cuneiform bones, metatarsal bones and their associated joints. Several disorders of the midfoot are most commonly seen in elderly patients but frequently go unrecognized.

Trauma to the midfoot, particularly dislocation of Lisfranc's joints, is often missed clinically and on roentgenographic studies. Several views, particularly oblique views, must be obtained to determine whether dislocation has occurred. Comparison views of the normal side are also helpful in making the diagnosis. Fractures of the metatarsal bones may also go unrecognized and are occasionally missed on roentgenograms. Although stress fractures occur more frequently in young patients, elderly patients with severe osteoporosis can present with stress fractures of the metatarsal bones, particularly of the third and fourth metatarsal shafts, and a bone scan may be necessary for making the diagnosis. Management of a metatarsal fracture consists of elevation of the involved limb, followed by use of cast or a wooden shoe until the patient is comfortable. Dislocation of a Lisfranc's joint is managed by closed or open reduction and internal fixation to prevent further deformity.

Another traumatic problem of the midfoot, recently recognized, involves rupture of the posterior tibial tendon (4). This tendon passes just below the medial malleolus and attaches to the tarsal navicular bone.

In addition to inverting the foot, the posterior tibial tendon stabilizes the midfoot on single stance and maintains the longitudinal arch. Patients with a rupture of the posterior tibial tendon describe progressive planovalgus (flatfoot deformity) and show swelling along the medial side of the foot. There may be a history of trauma. The abnormality usually progresses gradually over several months.

Rupture of the posterior tibial tendon can be easily diagnosed if it is kept in mind. There is an obvious flatfoot deformity in the involved limb. There is also weakness of the tendon, as demonstrated by single-toe raising. Also, when standing behind the patient and looking at the feet, the clinician notes extension of the forefoot in the lateral direction, which is commonly known as the "too many toes sign" (Figure 7.1). In most cases, the fourth or fifth toe is involved. With rupture of the tendon, the third or second toe may be affected, resulting in the too many toes sign. Arthritis and instability of the subtalar joint may be caused by rupture of the tendon. The rupture is probably related to chronic degeneration of the tendon. The rupture may occur at the point of attachment of the tendon to the navicular bone or within the tendon. Before such a rupture takes place, there may be signs of inflammation and tendinitis in the sheath of the posterior tibial tendon. These signs can be relieved by immobilization in a walking cast. However, once the tendon has ruptured, it must be repaired surgically to maintain adequate alignment of the forefoot. Primary repair or interposition of another tendon may be required. If there is progressive degenerative arthritis, fusion is the only management option.

Planovalgus is not always caused by rupture of the posterior tibial tendon. If the condition is bilateral, it is most likely congenital. Patients with extremely high arches may suffer from a neurologic disorder, such as Charcot-Marie-

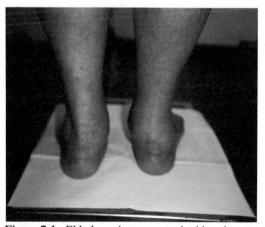

Figure 7.1. Elderly patient presented with a three-month history of progressive flatfoot deformity of her right foot. No history of trauma could be elicited, but the patient did note swelling and pain along the medial aspect of her foot and ankle prior to the onset of the flat foot.

This illustration demonstrates the lateral placement of the toes on the right ("too many toes") foot as compared to the left. There was also a weakness on the single toe rise of the foot, suggesting a rupture of the tibialis-posterior tendon. This was confirmed during surgical exploration.

Tooth disease, and diagnostic studies, including electromyograms, may be needed. In patients with hyperpronation of the forefoot, pain may develop along the medial side of the knee after prolonged walking. The pain can be relieved by use of an orthosis or a longitudinal arch support that prevents the hyperpronation. Knee symptoms usually resolve within two or three weeks after placement of the orthosis.

The base of the fifth metatarsal bone can be fractured by an inversion injury. The peroneus brevis tendon attaches to the proximal portion of the fifth metatarsal bone. After an inversion injury, a portion of this bone may be avulsed. Management consists of immobilization for four to six weeks.

Other disorders of the midfoot include acute bacterial infection and chronic infection, such as tuberculosis. In diabetic patients, Charcot's foot is often misdiagnosed as osteomyelitis. Careful inspection of roentgenograms permits differentiation between the two conditions. In Charcot's foot, there is destruction of the joints and bones; however, there also is obvious evidence of new bone formation. The latter finding is not observed in osteomyelitis. Most patients with Charcot's foot present with swelling and erythema but do not have a history of infection or trauma. Portions of the feet are anesthetic as a consequence of the diabetic peripheral neuropathy. In diabetic patients, Charcot's foot may also develop after an elective foot operation. Management initially involves immobilization in a well-padded cast and progressive ambulation. Within six to eight weeks, solidification of the bones may permit ambulation in a modified custom shoe. The prognosis for such patients is still poor, and those with diffuse foot involvement may eventually have to undergo amputation. Again, it is extremely important to differentiate Charcot's foot from osteomyelitis to avoid excessive use of antibiotics.

THE FOREFOOT

The forefoot includes the matatarso phalangeal joints and all structures distal to these joints.

On initial examination, most skin irritation and ulceration are found in the forefoot. Nail deformities may be the result of progressive changes (ram's horn nail) or chronic fungal infection. With ram's horn nail (onychogryposis), sanding does not correct the problem, so avulsion of the nail and ablation of the matrix may be necessary. This procedure prevents further deformity and allows easier skin care. In patients with chronic fungal infection, the use of a topical ointment and medication often does not resolve the problem. Oral administration of antifungal agents has been tried, in many cases with unsatisfactory results. In patients with brittle nails and breakage as a result of fungal infection, it is recommended that the nail be avulsed and the matrix ablated to eliminate the infection.

In patients who have difficulty trimming their nails, avulsion of the nail and ablation of the matrix permit easier care. Chronic cases of ingrown toenails should be managed in a similar manner. Oral administration of a broad-spectrum antibiotic is helpful in managing cellulitis in patients with acute infection.

Soft-tissue abnormalities of the forefoot also include hard and soft corns. Hard corns are usually related to the development of a bony prominence and irritation of the skin as a result of wearing improper shoes or from toes rubbing together. In many cases, corns can be managed by placing pads over the affected area and stretching the shoe. Surgical removal of a corn without partial resection of the underlying bone does not correct the problem. Over-the-counter ''corn plasters'' are of little benefit.

Soft corns, which usually develop at the base of the toe or in the web spaces, are related to irritation. Again, the bony prominence must be removed to correct the problem. Fungal infection of the web spaces can be managed with the use of a topical fungicide and better-fitting shoes.

Patients with splayfoot have difficulty finding appropriate footwear and thus often suffer from irritation over the metatarsophalangeal joints, especially those of the great and fifth toes. The irritated joints are commonly referred to as bunions or tailor's bunionettes (Figure 7.2). If appropriate footwear cannot be obtained, removal of the bony exostosis may be necessary. Plantar calluses are usually related to subluxation of the heads of the metatarsal bones and inadequate soft-tissue padding on the plantar surface of the foot. Causes include muscle imbalance related to a neurologic disorder (e.g., Charcot-Marie-Tooth disease), stroke, inflammatory arthritides of the metatarsophalangeal joints, particularly rheumatoid arthritis, and progressive biomechanical changes in the foot (Figure 7.3 a & b). In most cases, the calluses are located under the heads of the second, third and fourth metatarsal bones (Figure 7.4). In patients with extreme shortening of the first metatarsal bones (Morton's foot), calluses frequently develop under the heads of the second metatarsal bones as a result of a shift in the bearing of weight from the first to the second metatarsal bones.

In most cases, the symptoms can be relieved by paring the calluses with a sharp blade, and inserting a support device, such as a metatarsal pad proximal

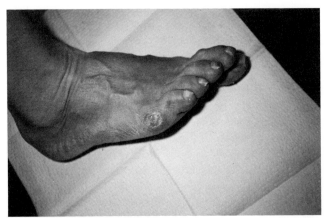

Figure 7.2. Tailor's bunion resulting from chronic skin irritation related to inadequate width of the shoe.

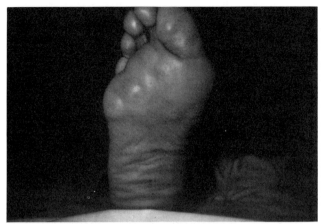

Figure 7.3a. Plantar hyperkeratoses of the foot as a result of plantar subluxation of the metatarsal heads.

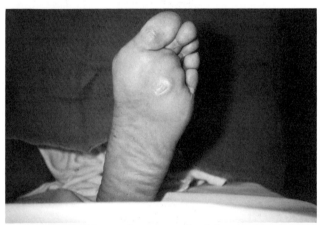

Figure 7.3b. In this case it was a result of rheumatoid arthritis.

to the heads of the metatarsal bones, to relieve pressure over the bony prominences. In the author's experience, orthopedic felt is an ideal pad because it does not collapse when weight is borne, is inexpensive and is easy to use. Hard rubber pads are uncomfortable and do not provide adequate relief of pressure. Over-the-counter pads are usually made of foam rubber and collapse immediately when weight is borne. In occasional cases, metatarsal bars are placed on the bottom of the shoe; however, if a patient has to climb stairs, the bars frequently get caught, predisposing to falls. The use of metatarsal bars should be avoided in elderly patients. Inserts made of a plastizote material may decrease pressure over the heads of the involved metatarsal bones. The material can be heated, and digital pressure at the appropriate level produces

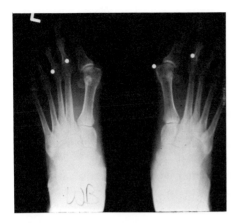

Figure 7.4. Lead markers placed on hyperkeratotic areas of the foot in order to locate the exact metatarsal heads which are involved.

an impression in the plastizote that relieves pressure over the heads of the metatarsal bones. Custom shoes are needed only if a patient has a number of deformities. Jogging shoes often provide the best fit and the most support for elderly patients. Such shoes allow for various widths in the toe box to prevent deformity, are lightweight and provide good support.

Breakdown of the skin beneath a callus may lead to the development of an ulcer and, possibly chronic infection. In such cases, active debridement with partial resection of the head of the metatarsal bone is required. In patients with recalcitrant calluses, surgical elevation or removal of the heads of the involved metatarsal bones may be necessary. However, this form of management may provoke the development of a transfer lesion, a possibility that necessitates the use of care during the surgical procedure.

A grading system has been developed for diabetic patients who have ulcers or infection of the foot. A grade I lesion is a simple callus with no or minimal evidence of ulceration. In a grade II lesion, there is an ulcer through the skin and subcutaneous tissue. A grade III lesion involves severe infection of the deeper structures of the foot. In a grade IV lesion, there is gangrene in a portion of the foot. Last, a grade V lesion is manifested by gangrene of the entire foot. Most grade I lesions can be managed by use of appropriate footwear. Grade II and III lesions require active debridement and, possibly resection of the heads of the metatarsal bones or partial ray amputation to save the remainder of the foot. Systemic administration of an antibiotic does not resolve the infection, and surgical debridement is necessary. In grade IV and V lesions, amputation may be the only management option. Early aggressive management of infection in a diabetic patient may allow part of the foot to be saved for a prolonged period. However, once the deep soft tissues and other structures are involved, local management is extremely difficult.

Disorders of the metatarsophalangeal joints also include inflammatory and degenerative arthritides and gout. Tophi can develop in elderly women in the metatarsophalangeal joints of the lesser toes and great toe. Occasionally encountered are draining lesions, which are often misdiagnosed as evidence of chronic infection. The diagnosis relies on microscopy to demonstrate uric acid crystals in the drainage material. A common condition is degenerative arthritis of the metatarsophalangeal joint of the great toe, which leads to hallux rigidus. Active and passive range of motion of the metatarsophalangeal joint is markedly limited. An effusion may be observed. Most cases can be managed with conservative measures, including placement of an orthosis with an extension over the first metatarsophalangeal joint, use of an anti-inflammatory agent and, occasionally, intra-articular injection of a corticosteroid. In severe cases with marked limitation of joint motion, debridement, resection arthroplasty or implant arthroplasty with a Silastic hinge implant may be necessary. The double-hinge Silastic implants used in the management of hallux rigidus have been effective in relieving pain and improving ambulation. Breakage of the implant, infection and silicone synovitis are potential complications. Degenerative arthritis of the metatarsophalangeal joints of the lesser toes is encountered infrequently, except in cases of trauma. As was noted previously, gout may occur in the lesser toe joints, as may inflammatory arthritides, such as rheumatoid arthritis. In some cases, subluxation of the phalanx dorsally worsens the deformity of the toes. Management consists of modification of footwear or, in severe cases, surgical correction.

Other problems of the great toe are hallux valgus and recurrent bunions. Surgical management of bunions is generally reserved for patients with chronic pain who are unable to obtain properly fitting footwear. In most cases, shoes can be stretched over a bunion to provide adequate support and alleviate chronic pain. The choice of surgical therapy depends on the degree of bony deformity, the severity of arthritis and the extent of soft-tissue contracture. In patients with adequate peripheral circulation, age is not a contraindication for surgical intervention if the foot problem markedly limits ambulation and activities of daily living.

Deformities of the forefoot also include hammer toe, claw toe and an overlapping second toe. In most cases, these deformities are related to biomechanical changes in the foot, except perhaps for claw toe, which may result from neurologic impairment. In a hammer toe, there is flexion of the proximal interphalangeal joint, but the distal interphalangeal joint is normal. By contrast, in a claw toe, there is flexion of both joints. Conservative management consists of placement of pads over the appropriate sites or modification of footwear. If conservative management is unsuccessful, surgical correction is necessary. An overlapping toe can also be corrected by the use of pads, and surgical management may be required only in patients with chronic pain or ulcers related to irritation of bone.

Pain and paresthesias in the distal portions of the toes are caused by a variety of neurologic lesions. Peripheral neuropathy and other proximal neurologic lesions were discussed earlier in this chapter. Occasional cases are caused by neuroma in the web spaces. The typical location is between the third and fourth toes, a condition known as Morton's neuroma. Patients present with pain and paresthesias, usually after wearing a closed shoe. These symptoms are relieved with rest and elevation of the foot; rubbing of the toes frequently helps restore sensation.

Clinical findings include pain elicited on lateral compression of the involved metatarsal bones and tenderness on direct palpation of the web space. Rarely does a patient have more than one neuroma on one foot. The symptoms are usually relieved by injection of a corticosteroid and local instillation of an anesthetic into the web spaces. If the symptoms persist, removal of the neuroma is indicated. Metatarsalgia or synovitis of the metatarsophalangeal joints may be accompanied by symptoms similar to those of neuroma, often making the diagnosis difficult. In most cases, local administration of an anesthetic helps distinguish between joint symptoms and those of web-space neuroma.

Some patients have pain and swelling in the metatarsophalangeal joints of the lesser toes. Roentgenograms show no evidence of bony or arthritic problems. The diagnosis is usually metatarsalgia or capsulitis syndrome. The etiologic basis of these disorders remains unclear; however, it appears that patients with recurrent metatarsalgia and synovitis in the lesser toes may have disruption of the plantar plate. The disruption may worsen the synovitis; occasionally, further examination of the joints shows effusion and inflammation of the synovium. Surgical examination usually demonstrates a tear within the plantar plate. In a few cases, there is a flap type of injury to the plate that causes the plate to impinge on the metatarsophalangeal joint, resulting in "locking" or "clicking" sensations. The diagnosis is often difficult; however, local injection of an anesthetic into the joint helps delineate the problem. In recurrent cases, exploration of the joint with partial resection of the plate may be required to prevent progressive changes.

One would be remiss in discussing problems of the foot without touching on blood flow in the foot. The evaluation of peripheral vascular disease includes sequential measurements of blood pressure and, possibly angiography. In cases in which amputation is being considered, xenon flow studies are extremely helpful in determining blood supply to the soft tissues and skin and are the most accurate studies for predicting whether a wound will heal after surgical intervention. Most surgeons advocate removal of as little tissue as possible, but it appears that elderly patients can achieve fairly good function and do better with a below-knee amputation than with a more-distal amputation.

Energetic rehabilitation after amputation should not be reserved for only young patients. Many elderly patients who undergo amputation, including bilateral amputees, regain the ability to ambulate after participating in a vigorous program of physical therapy. In most cases, such therapy involves the placement of a prosthesis immediately after operation to permit ambulation as quickly as is feasible. It is less likely that ambulation will be restored after above-knee amputations because greater expenditure of energy is required for using an above-knee prosthesis. However, active elderly patients may regain this ability even with such a device.

The decision regarding amputation should be based on a patient's ambulatory capabilities and on concern for adequate healing.

In summary, foot disorders are commonly encountered in elderly patients. A careful evaluation of the feet and ankles should be part of the physical examination. Of the many foot disorders, most can be managed by modification of footwear or the use of appropriate pads or other devices. In recalcitrant cases, surgical management should be considered regardless of a patient's age.

REFERENCES

1. Carter, S.A. The relationship of distal systolic pressures to healing of skin lesions in limbs with arterial occlusive disease with special reference to diabetes mellitus. *Scand. J. Clin. Lab. Invest. Suppl.* 31(124):239–243, 1973.
2. Gibbons, G.W., Wheelock, F.C., Siembieda, C., Hoar, C.S., Rowbotham, J.L., and Persson, A.B. Noninvasive prediction of amputation level in diabetic patients. *Arch. Surg.* (Chicago) 114:1253–1257, 1979.
3. Wagner, F.W., Jr., and Buggs, H. Use of Doppler ultrasound in determining healing levels in diabetic dysvascular lower extremity problems, in Bergan, J.J., and Yao, J.S.T. (eds.): *Gangrene and Severe Ischemia of the Lower Extremities.* New York, Grune & Stratton, 1978, pp. 131–138.
4. Johnson, K. Tibialis posterior tendon rupture. *Clin. Orthop. Relat. Res.* 177:140–147, 1983.

Chapter 8

L. Gregory Pawlson
Carole Bernstein Lewis

Dysmobility

We will use the word dysmobility as a general term to denote any problem relating to getting from one place to another. The problem can range from difficulty transferring from bed to chair to problems associated with driving a motor vehicle. Table 8.1 lists a number of problems that can be subsumed under this term. Community surveys of the elderly reveal that more than 15 percent of people over age 65 have some type of mobility problem, not including those relating to the use of public transportation or driving. Nearly 85 percent of people confined to nursing homes have some major problem with mobility. However, even these striking figures seem to underestimate the problem because many elderly people consider dysmobility to be a normal concomitant of aging and therefore may not report it as a problem.

DIAGNOSIS

The history can offer clues to emerging problems before they have produced marked functional impairment. For example, a history of slips and near-falls while using public transportation may be a prelude to a fall that produces a hip fracture or an elderly patient's withdrawal from social interactions due to a mobility problem. A change in a patient's usual activity pattern can be an important manifestation of dysmobility. Other inquiries as to a patient's ability to drive, use public transportation, climb steps and walk on a level surface are important. Also helpful are questions concerning a fear of falling. Several studies have shown that a fear of falling may be an important determinant of mobility. Obviously, symptoms relating to specific diseases, such as osteoarthritis or Parkinson's disease, should be explored in full. Table 8.2 lists other questions that can help define dysmobility.

Perhaps the most important element in characterizing dysmobility is the physical examination. With the exception of auscultation or use of an electrocardiogram to characterize heart disease, there is little agreement in most textbooks about which direct measurements of mobility should be included in the physical exami-

TABLE 8.1   Types of Dysmobility

Transferring
  Bed to chair to commode
  Standing or sitting to bathtub
  Bed to standing
  Standing to chair
Self-propelling a wheelchair
Walking
  Level surface
  Incline
  Stairs: two or three steps
  Stairs: 10 or more steps
Using public transportation
Driving a car

TABLE 8.2   History

Frequency of walks/trips outside the house
Frequency of interaction with family/friends
Recent motor vehicle accidents
Difficulty using buses, subway or taxis
Falls, slips or near-falls
Trauma (bruises, fractures, lacerations)
Stated ability to walk, climb stairs or transfer

nation of elderly patients. However, the examination should include traditional elements, such as observation of gait and station, as well as a functional assessment of mobility in most cases. A carefully planned observation of a patient entering the examination room or answering the door at home can serve as a screening test for many forms of dysmobility (Table 8.3). A description of any abnormality of gait along with the ease of turning and transferring from the standing to the sitting position and to the standing position again can easily and quickly be accomplished by such careful observation. If any question of difficulty arises, the patient should undergo the full examination and assessment

TABLE 8.3   Routine Physical Examination

Functional assessment of gait and transfers: careful, planned observation of patient walking across room (10 feet or more), turning around, sitting down in and getting up from chair and resuming walk.

Gait	Frequency, height, length and symmetry of steps, balance, coordination, associative movements
	Abnormalities: shuffling, waddling, hesitancy, ataxia, acceleration (festinating), circumduction, staggering, foot slapping, short steps, wide base
Transfers	Coordination, use of arms, resumption of walking
	Abnormalities: fall or near-fall into chair, more than one attempt to get out of chair, primary use of arms, hesitancy or unsteadiness in resumption of gait

TABLE 8.4 More Thorough Physical
Examination When Dysmobility Suspected

Range of motion of weight-bearing joints
Examination of weight-bearing joints for deformity
Strength of legs
Romberg test
Heel to shin test
Position, touch and pain sensation in legs
Ankle reflex, Babinski's reflex
Mental status examination
Visual acuity test

outlined in Tables 8.4 and 8.5. Timed walk or timed transfer is especially useful in assessing progress or decline of a patient's mobility over time. Testing a patient for the ability to climb two or three steps is relevant to the use of public transportation, while the ability to climb a flight of stairs can be important to persons who reside in or visit buildings with stairs and no elevators.

RISK FACTORS

Dysmobility is obviously a symptom or nonspecific problem rather than a disease or specific entity. As is often the case with nonspecific problems in elderly patients, the causes of dysmobility can be multifactorial. In other words, dysmobility is frequently the result of the interaction of several risk factors. A brief discussion of some common risk factors for dysmobility in the elderly follows; additional risk factors are listed in Table 8.6.

Chronic Arthritis

Any type of chronic arthritis that involves the back or legs can result in problems with mobility. Osteoarthritis, a degenerative joint disease that commonly afflicts the elderly, usually involves the large weight-bearing joints, such as the knees or hips, that are important in walking. Apart from any joint deformity, the pain from chronic arthritis alone can be a major factor in producing a vicious cycle of pain leading to less exercise, to contractures and decreased strength and to more pain with any type of movement. In addition, most types of chronic arthritis can produce secondary changes in joints due to abnormal stresses placed on the joints during walking. Many secondary problems become manifest as a

TABLE 8.5 Physical Examination: Functional Assessment Tests

Timed walk (e.g., 25 feet)
Two steps up and down
Time to climb stairs (12 or more steps)
Ability to reach above head (or into cabinet) and maintain balance
Ability to bend down to pick up object on floor

TABLE 8.6 Additional Risk Factors
for Dysmobility in the Elderly

Visual changes
  Cataracts
  Macular degeneration
Chronic obstructive pulmonary disease
Chronic alcoholism
Middle-ear disease
  Meniere's disease
  Labyrinthine vertigo
Postural hypotension
Diabetes
  Autonomic neuropathy
  Peripheral neuropathy
  Visual loss
Atherosclerotic cardiovascular disease
  Angina
  Claudication
Pernicious anemia
Severe malnutrition

person ages. Arthritis that involves the small joints of the feet can also have a profound effect on mobility. Most especially, the involvement of the first metatarsophalangeal joint in patients with arthritis or deformity can produce marked abnormalities of gait.

Local Disorders of the Feet and Toes

Such disorders as flat feet, metatarsalgia and bunions and hammer toe deformity, which may be relatively well tolerated by young adults, can, when combined with other risk factors or the normal physiologic process of aging, produce marked dysmobility. In many instances, the conditions are slowly progressive and do not produce major functional impairment until relatively advanced age. Other local foot problems, such as corns, calluses and ingrown toenails, are sometimes so severe that they lead to problems with gait in elderly persons, especially when poor vision or loss of function of the arms, for example, makes foot care impossible. Community surveys of the health problems of the elderly have revealed that foot problems are the most common unmet health need perceived by such people.

Degenerative Neurologic Diseases

DEMENTIA

In the middle stages of chronic progressive dementia and at virtually any stage of dementia secondary to multiple cortical infarcts, a disturbance of gait may become a serious problem. A number of aspects of dementia appear to be related to abnormalities of gait, including loss of motivation for walking, an ataxia of gait and reduced ability to use assistive devices, loss of cognizance of safety factors and reduced ability to participate in gait training secondary to the cognitive deficit. The neurologic changes responsible for the decline in mobility include loss of visuospatial skills, coordination, motor planning and balance.

NORMAL-PRESSURE HYDROCEPHALUS
Although relatively uncommon, normal-pressure hydrocephalus, with its triad of poor bladder control, slow and infrequent speech with some cognitive dysfunction and a slow, wide-based, clumsy, shuffling gait, is of importance because of the potential for control or reversal of the symptoms. In addition to this triad, the syndrome is often accompanied by abnormal reflexes (grasp, snout, plantar) and frequent falls. Symptoms progress relatively rapidly (over a few months). The diagnosis is suggested by computerized tomogram that shows dilatation of the ventricles out of proportion to overall atrophy and by a cisterno-gram that demonstrates reflux into the ventricles and delayed cerebral diffusion. If the syndrome is diagnosed in its early stages, improvement can be expected with ventriculoatrial shunting and intensive rehabilitation efforts.

PARKINSON'S DISEASE
The rigidity, hypokinesis, postural hypotension and loss of balance often associated with Parkinson's disease cause a number of abnormalities of gait that can lead to dysmobility. The classical parkinsonian gait of small, hesitant steps is largely the result of difficulty with making the corrections of balance and coordination that are needed to produce a smooth, steady gait. Also characteristics of Parkinson's disease are the classical festinating gait, in which a patient virtually runs to avoid falling forward, and a slowness in initiating new movements, including transfers. Although muscle strength is relatively unaffected in the early stages, the disturbance of gait often leads to a reduction in overall exercise and, subsequently to a marked loss of strength. Finally, perhaps 30 percent of patients with longstanding Parkinson's disease suffer from dementia, which imposes an additional burden on a patient's efforts to maintain mobility.

Atherosclerotic Cardiovascular Disease

STROKE
Obviously, weakness or paralysis of one or both legs has a profound effect on mobility. The classical spastic hemiplegic gait with its characteristic stiffness and circumduction is the most dramatic result of a stroke. Muscle strength, motor planning and coordination can also be adversely affected by a stroke. For example, a frontal-lobe stroke can give rise to an ataxia of gait similar to that seen in dementia. A small brain stem stroke can lead to the so-called

toppling gait, in which there is a sudden loss of balance and consequent falls. Difficulty with mobility, often in the form of falls, can also occur with transient ischemic attacks as a result of the onset of unilateral weakness or a so-called drop attack.

CORONARY AND PERIPHERAL VASCULAR DISEASE

Although the major manifestations of coronary-artery disease are not usually thought of in relation to mobility, this disease can have a profound effect on mobility. Obviously, angina or severe congestive heart failure can greatly restrict a person's mobility. Some people who are confined to wheelchairs became that way simply as an adversive reaction to angina or severe claudication. In addition, some people have strong beliefs that exercise is contraindicated by cardiovascular disease.

Age

It is often difficult to sort out the effects of physiologic aging from the effects produced by chronic diseases that are nearly universal in elderly people, such as osteoarthritis and cardiovascular disease. The so-called senile gait, which consists of slow, hesitant, uncertain steps with a flexed posture and a loss of associative movements, can occur with aging alone but is accelerated by such diseases as osteoarthritis and Parkinson's disease. The slowing of reaction time and loss of muscle strength, coordination and motor planning that are inevitable with aging are relatively modest in degree but can in combination produce a marked effect on mobility. Careful assessment of a patient over time should help delineate most independent risk factors from the aging process.

Disuse

A major contributing factor to the loss of mobility often seen in the elderly is simply disuse. The present cohort of elderly people in their eighties and nineties believe that they are too old to participate in any type of exercise. Both aerobic (conditioning) exercise and flexibility (range-of-motion) exercise are important in maintaining mobility. Any intercurrent illness that necessitates bedrest for even a few days can result in a major loss of mobility due to loss of strength and cardiovascular deconditioning. With more prolonged bedrest, shortening of tendons and loss of muscle mass can have a profound effect on attempts to mobilize a patient.

CONSEQUENCES

A loss of mobility can lead to dramatic changes in a person's lifestyle and even severe depression. Dysmobility can interfere with an elderly's person's interaction with friends or family. It can also prevent participation in such activities as shopping, going to social events and attending church. It is important for clinicians to be able to recognize and suggest appropriate intervention in instances where dysmobility is a major factor contributing to a patient's loss of social interaction and depression. Fortunately, in many urban areas, there are a variety of transportation and escort services that may greatly improve the lifestyles of the elderly with severe mobility problems.

REHABILITATION TO MANAGEMENT

Obviously, the management of risk factors may greatly enhance mobility. However, in many cases, management must focus on the generic problem of dysmobility having a multifactorial basis. Sometimes, a relatively small adjustment or improvement in several risk factors relating to dysmobility can produce a relatively dramatic improvement. Although a diagnostic assessment has been suggested, it is usually necessary to perform further assessment before embarking on management. The focus of the therapeutic assessment is on further documentation of the current status of a patient and exploration of potential barriers to rehabilitation. In most instances, a rehabilitation professional, such as a physical therapist or physiatrist, should be involved in the assessment.

Although rehabilitation professionals are crucial in assessing, managing and modifying the environment to prevent immobility and improve mobility, primary-care physicians should have a clear understanding of the process. The rest of this chapter will discuss therapeutic assessments and interventions for mobility problems commonly seen in the elderly. After using the information presented in the previous section and in other chapters, the major causes and risk factors can be determined. At this point, a more detailed therapeutic assessment should be conducted for the purpose of setting up guidelines for a specific rehabilitation program.

The components of the therapeutic assessment are as follows:

1. Problem goals and history
2. Physical evaluation
3. Drugs
4. Psychologic evaluation
5. Mobility grade
6. Environment
7. Support system

In the problem goals and history section, a rehabilitation professional identifies the major reason a patient is coming for treatment. Once the reason has been determined, goals are set for specific outcomes after completion of the treatment regimen. During the history portion, the patient relates relevant information about the nature and duration of prior disabilities. An example of a typical interaction for this section of the evaluation form is as follows:

Dr. J: Hi Ms. Jones. I am going to ask you a few questions about why you are here. What would you say is your major problem?

Ms. J: I am unable to go up and down stairs.

Dr. J: How long have you had this problem?

Ms. J: I've been weak in my knees for a while—two years, but about six months ago, I fell down three steps.

Dr. J: Well, Ms. J, what would you like the outcome to be after you're done here?

Ms. J: I'd like to be able to walk up and down the stairs without falling and being out of breath.

The physical examination includes an evaluation of the integrity of the skin in areas predisposed to the development of pressure sores. The cardiopulmonary system can be assessed by determining the heart rate and blood pressure and looking for pathologic problems. Assessment of the musculoskeletal system includes an evaluation of leg motion and strength. Special attention should be given to the calf muscles, checking for stiffness of the plantar flexors (dorsiflexion should be at least 10 degrees, past neutral) and strength of the plantar flexors (normal strength allows a person to hop on one foot). The plantar flexors have an important role in providing safe propulsion while walking as well as in maintaining balance. Another muscle group that tends to show weakness and tightness in the elderly consists of the hip muscles. Finally, the feet deserve special consideration and should be checked for skin integrity and abnormalities that often restrict mobility. In the neurologic assessment, the leg reflexes, vibratory sense, proprioception, tremor, tone and sway pattern should be examined.

The psychologic assessment of mobility problems can be subjectively accomplished by asking questions about the four major categories. Specifically, the examiner can ask a patient about his or her fear of falling and desire to be mobile or can subjectively glean such information from other portions of the evaluation (i.e., the history). Several quick tools that can disclose dementia or depression can be given to the patient (i.e., the Mini Mental or the Beck Depression Inventory.

The drug section of the assessment simply lists the various prescribed and over-the-counter drugs but could also indicate the dosage of each medication.

The mobility section determines the patient's independence at each mobility level. Mobility can be graded from poor to normal with type of assistance (i.e., maximal assist of 2, to minimal assist of 1, to independent). These ratings can be used to evaluate bed, sitting, transfer and standing mobilities. The ratings can then be used as guidelines for monitoring the patient's progress through the rehabilitation program. Finally, a gait analysis can be performed by evaluating the trunk, hip, knee and ankle components of the gait cycle. In addition, gait-evaluation tools can supplement this section of the assessment (1,2).

An environmental assessment can truly be done only in the living environment; therefore, in an outpatient setting, cursory questioning is the best means of analysis. Areas to be noted are lighting, rugs and floors. Special considerations are:

A. Lighting
 1. Ensure adequacy
 2. Avoid dark to light contrast
B. Rugs
 1. Suggest nonskid
 2. Provide color contrast
C. Floors
 1. Minimize glare
 2. Design even, safe surfaces

The support system can be evaluated by asking the patient whom he or she lives with and who visits and provides assistance. This assessment is general. If specific deficiencies are noted, a more thorough evaluation can be conducted in any area.

The final section, miscellaneous, identifies other important aspects not noted earlier.

Use of a team approach for assessing mobility problems in the elderly is ideal; for managing mobility problems, it is essential. A physician, a nurse, a social worker, a pharmacist, an occupational therapist and a physical therapist can easily split up the assessment instrument and combine the necessary portions for treatment, or one well-trained member of the team can assess the patient and determine the appropriate treatment regimen to be used by each team member. The following management lists are for the various disciplines:

Physical Therapy
 GOALS
  Improve range of motion
  Improve strength
  Improve coordination
  Improve gait and balance
  Improve sitting, standing and transfers
  Teach the use of assistive ambulatory devices
  Modify activities to improve mobility and to relieve pain safely
 Interventions
  Exercise—active, passive and neuromuscular
  Soft-tissue manipulation
  Joint mobilization

Gait training and modification
Coordination and endurance training
Balance and transfer training
Environmental and ergometric training
Modalities to relieve pain and to increase strength and flexibility
Ambulatory aid training
Designing splints for legs

Occupational Therapy
GOALS
Improve functional independence
Improve perceptual and sensory function
Improve independence in activities of daily living
Improve problem-solving skills
Improve leisure skills
Interventions
Bed, transfer and wheelchair training
Providing splints
Training in activities of daily living (dressing, toileting, bathing, cooking and personal hygiene)
Environmental assessment
Exercise—active, passive and neuromuscular
Designing leisure activities (i.e., crafts)
Recommendations and training in use of assistive devices (i.e., reachers and grippers)
Recommendations and training in use of safety devices (i.e., grab bars and toilet seats)

Social Work
GOALS
Improve social support systems
Design interventions to enhance independence
Interventions
Family counseling
Individual counseling
Resource and referral for community services
Liaison to community and institutions

Nursing
GOALS
Improve overall functioning
Improve skin integrity
Improve functional ability
Improve general mobility

Interventions
    Drug administration
    Positioning
    Restorative care
    Continuous patient interaction
    Skin care
    Assistance in activities of daily living and transfers
    Safety modification and supervision
    Ongoing assessment

Pharmacy
    GOAL
        Improve drug usage
    Intervention
        Ongoing drug analysis

The remainder of this chapter will focus on assistive ambulatory aids, environmental safety assessments and specific exercises for mobility problems.

AMBULATORY AIDS

Eighty-seven percent of elderly people have no limitation to mobility; however, the remainder of the elderly population use a cane, crutch, walker or wheelchair or are bedridden (3). The chart that follows gives indications, assessments, contraindications and special instructions.

Crutches are not generally recommended for elderly patients because they are difficult to manipulate and exert undue pressure in the axilla if a patient has inadequate strength in the affected arm. In addition, crutches necessitate better balance if three-point gait is used.

Ambulatory aids should always be considered when a patient relates a history of a decreased ability to ambulate that interferes with function. In addition, distance walked is important. One study cited distances ambulated to common locations frequented by the elderly and patients' abilities to walk such distances (4). This study revealed major differences in patients' ambulatory abilities, speed of walking and ability to negotiate curb heights. Rehabilitation professionals need to further document the need to intervene to improve elderly patients' functional ambulation distance, walking speed and step heights so that such patients are truly independent in the community.

Environmental Safety Assessment

Independent, safe mobility depends on a safe environment. *The Sixth Sense* (5), a program of the National Council on Aging, provides a form useful for this purpose. This form was designed for the home environment but can easily be adapted for use in nursing homes.

Ambulatory Aids

	CANE	WHEELED WALKER	WHEELCHAIR
Indication	1. Leg weakness 2. Slight balance problems 3. Slight endurance problems 4. Pain on weight bearing 5. Endurance complications 6. Arm weakness	1. Leg weakness 2. Nonweight bearing one limb 3. Partial weight bearing one limb 4. Gait instability one limb 5. Joint pain	1. Severe leg weakness 2. Severe balance and coordination problems 3. Severe endurance problems 4. Upper-body complications 5. Severe joint pain
Assessment	Patient stands and cane is measured six inches from side and elbow is bent to 20 degrees	Patient stands and walker is measured with hands on grip and elbows bent to 20 degrees	Measurement: Seat width: hip width plus one inch on each side Seat depth: femur less three inches Seat back height: $\simeq$ 18 inches depending on support needed Floor to seat height: $\simeq$ 19 inches; hemi chairs: 17 inches
Contraindication	If patient appears unsafe with trial cane	If patient is too weak to lift walker (use wheeled walker)	Last choice because dependence on wheelchair can add to bedrest deconditioning
Special instructions	1. Use cane when pain occurs 2. Use cane for long trips 3. Use cane when feeling unstable 4. Do not elevate shoulder when using 5. Use with uninvolved arm 6. Do not slouch over cane	Specific safety instructions for rising to and sitting down from walker	Specific transfer-training instructions Specific safety instructions Low-back supports (rolled towels) for patients with flat backs and low-back pain

Sample Mobility Assessment

Name _____ Date _____
Functional Problem _____
Goals _____
History _____
_____

Physical Evaluation _____
   Skin _____
   Cardiopulmonary BP _____ HR _____
    Pathology _____
   Musculoskeletal
    ROM _____
    STR _____
    FEET _____
   Neurologic
    Reflexes _____ Proprioception _____
    Vibration _____ Sway _____
    Tremor _____ Tone _____
   Psychologic
    Motivation _____ Depression _____
    Dementia _____ Falling Fear _____
   Drugs
    Prescribed _____ OTC _____
   Environment _____
   Mobility Grade
    Bed _____ Sitting _____
    Transfer _____ Wheelchair _____
    Standing _____
    Gait _____
   Support System _____
   MISC _____

Exercise

Various interventions have proved successful in managing balance problems. For the backward thrusting commonly seen during transferring and ambulating, the following interventions may help:

1. Prone positioning for 15 to 20 minutes before transferring or ambulating.
2. Parasympathetic techniques
   a. Soft talk
   b. Gentle stroking as long as three minutes
   c. Midline touch
3. Gait training and facilitating from the front.

For an unsteady gait, hip exercises and plantar flexion exercises are helpful. In addition, various hints for balance are helpful.

Balance Hints

1. Maintain adequate base of support. (Stand with feet slightly apart.)
2. Lower center of gravity when greater stability needed. (Crouch when a fall is imminent.)
3. Keep the line of gravity within the base of support. (Stand with proper body alignment.)
4. Widen base of support in direction of force. (Lean into the wind.)
5. Increase friction between body and supporting surface for better stability. (Wear rubber-sole shoes for better gripping action.)
6. Maintain adequate strength to provide necessary force to regain balance after unexpected loss. (Maintain leg strength.)
7. Focus vision on stationary objects rather than on moving objects.
8. Mental practice.

Hip exercises include standing hip circles (the hula) and hip thrusts (to the side, forward and back). Plantar flexion exercises include toe ups and calf stretches. These exercises yield the best results if they are done at least 10 times, three times per day.

For painful knees, gentle stretching, strengthening and loosening exercises can provide positive results. The exercise programs that follow are used for patients with painful knees.

Traditional Exercise Program

1. Quad set exercise
   A. Tighten the muscles on top of the thigh as much as possible and hold.
      Hint: It will help with this and other exercises if, while you tighten, you
      a. Pull the toes back
      b. Push the back of the knee down to the floor
      c. Try to push out and up through the heel.
   B. Pull 10 seconds, trying every second to pull even tighter.
      Relax 10 seconds.
      Bend the knee three times as in No. 3.
2. Bend the knee toward the bottom, sliding the heel on the floor or the bed, three times between each of the above sets.
3. Drake exercise
   A. Tighten the muscles on top of the thigh as in exercise No. 2 and hold for two seconds.
   B. Lift the entire thigh about six inches as one solid unit and hold in the air for two seconds.
   C. Still keeping the muscles tight, bring the leg back to the floor or the bed, and tighten even harder for two seconds longer.
   D. Relax.
   E. Repeat 10 times, bending the knees three times as in No. 3. Relax and do 10 more repetitions.
      This exercise is easy if you concentrate. If you do not tighten the knee muscles to their absolute maximum, you are not gaining much benefit from the Drake exercise. If you have trouble, stop and rest a moment, after giving it one more try with more concentration.
4. Short-arc extension
   A. Bend the knee and place a hard object under it to hold it at a height of about six inches.

B. Raise the lower leg until the knee is as straight as possible, and do a quad set. Again, use all the hints in No. 1 (pull the toes back, push down on the block, push out and up through the heel).

C. Pull 10 seconds, trying every second to pull tighter. Relax for 10 seconds. Repeat for two sets of 10 repetitions, resting between sets and doing exercise No. 3 between sets.

5. Hamstring exercise
   A. Lying on the stomach, bend one knee, bringing the foot toward the posterior side of the thigh.
   B. Repeat 10 times. Relax and do 10 more repetitions.

6. Tow-raise exercise
   A. While standing up straight with feet together, turn the heels out slightly so that you are now standing a bit pigeon-toed.
   B. Raise up and down on the toes, making sure to go both ways as far as possible. Try to keep your weight distributed equally on both legs.
   C. Repeat 25 times, the above exercise.
   D. Facing the wall and keeping the heels flat, lean into the wall so that you feel a stretch in the calf muscles. Hold for 30 seconds.
   E. Do 25 more toes ups and then one more calf stretch on each side.

Coke-Bottle Exercise
1. Sit comfortably in a chair.
2. Place a Coke bottle under one foot.
3. Gently roll foot back and forth.
   This exercise can be done while watching television, sitting at a bridge game and so on. Begin with two to three minutes and build to 10 to 20 minutes.

Finally, visualization can help patients with balance problems. The following sample transcript can be used to improve balance (6).

Transcript

"Now think about balancing. Remember what it was like to play balancing games as a child. Remember how easy it was to stand on one leg. Remember how long you could balance playing hopscotch. Remember how easy and fun it was to walk along a thin wall."

"Think about your balance now. Realize that the balance you had as a child is still yours. You can balance; you just need to practice and to remind yourself of how easy it can be."

"As you stand on one leg, see yourself as a tall oak tree. Feel the support of the roots beneath you. Feel your arms like branches, reaching out to the sky, helping to support you in the air. Enjoy the feeling of standing calm and still in the wind."

"See a large, brightly colored bird. Imagine you are that bird. You have long, strong legs. You lift up one leg and begin to balance. Feel how securely you stand on one leg with the other tucked comfortably up beneath you" (6).

Exercises for the feet can be extremely beneficial for sore, weak and inflexible feet. Such exercises are easy to do, but they need to be pursued slowly. Some common exercises are:

1. Toe curls
2. Toe extensions
3. Toe spreads
4. Ankle bends
5. Ankle circles

Specific strengthening and stretching exercises can be beneficial for specific problems and should be encouraged, remembering that elderly persons need longer exercise sessions and longer exercise regimens (several weeks longer than young persons doing the exercises). Therefore, home exercise programs and periodic rechecks on progress are important aspects of such programs.

CONCLUSION

Independent mobility is an important goal for many elderly people. Creativity in assessment and interventions can enhance results and help patients achieve and maintain independence.

REFERENCES

1. Nelson, A.J. Functional ambulation profile. *Phys. Ther.* 54(10):1059–1065, 1974.
2. Parker, K.S., Zablotny, C.M., and Jordan, C. Analysis and management of hemiplegic gait dysfunction: Current concepts, in *Stroke Rehabilitation: State of the Art 1984*. Downey, Calif., Rancho Los Amigos Medical Center, 1984, pp. 33–47.
3. U.S. Senate Special Committee on Aging and the American Association of Retired Persons. *Aging America: Trends and Projection 1984*.
4. Lerner-Frankel, M., Vargus, S., and Brown, M.B. Functional community ambulation: What are your criteria. *Clin. Manage.* 6(2):72–86, 1985.
5. National Council on Aging. *The Sixth Sense,* 1985.
6. Fansler, C., Poff, C., and Shepard, K. Effects of mental practice on balance in elderly women. *Phys. Ther.* 65(9):1332–1338, 1985.

SUGGESTED READINGS

Guimavair, R.M., and Isaacs, B. Characteristics of gait in old people who fall. *Int. Rehabil. Med.* 2:177–180, 1980. A careful study of the characteristics of gait in a group of elderly persons who fell and in elderly persons who had not fallen. The slow, short, wide-based, variable gait is documented as a significant risk factor.

Pawlson, L.G., Goodwin, M., Keith, K. Wheelchair use by ambulatory nursing home residents. *J. Amer. Geriatr, Soc.* 34(12):860–864, 1986.

Sabin, T.D. Biological aspects of falls and mobility limitations in the elderly. *J. Amer. Geriatr. Soc.* 30:51–58, 1982. A thorough discussion of the pathophysiologic aspects of disturbances in gait in the elderly. Although the major emphasis is on such aspects, there is much clinically useful information in the article.

Tinetti, M.E. Performance oriented assessment of mobility problems in elderly patients. *J. Amer. Geriatr. Soc.* 34:119–126, 1986. An excellent review of the assessments needed to characterize dysmobility in elderly persons.

Index

Page numbers in italics refer to figures and tables.

of rotator cuffs, 48
for shoulder pain, 43–44
Raynaud's phenomenon, 66
Redness, inflammation and, 98–99
Reflex dystrophy, shoulder pain and, 54
Reiter's syndrome, lower back pain and, 25–27
Retrocalcaneal bursitis, Achilles tendinitis confused with, 115
Rheumatism, soft-tissue types, 12
Rheumatoid arthritis, *19*
    age onset for, 4
    in ankles, 114
    cervical spine lesions in, 19–21
    in hands and wrists, 64–65
    in knees, 105–109
    metacarpophalangeal joints involved in, 10
    osteoarthritis compared with, 1
    presentations of, 64–65
    stenosing tenosynovitis in, 62
    surgical management of, 65
    variable presentation of, 4
Rheumatoid synovitis, hydrocortisone to treat, 107
Rheumatologists, v–vi
Roentgenographic studies, 10, 11
    ankylosing spondylitis and Forestier's disease distinguished using, 30
    for lower back pain, 24–25
    predictive value of, 4
    of seronegative arthropathies, 65
Rotator cuff tendons, 41
    arthography in diagnosis of tears in, 44
    lesions of, 45–46
    ruptures of, 48

S
Sarcoidosis, 73
Scaphoid bone, 79
Scleroderma, 66
Sclerosis, at femur, 89
Sensory deficits, neurogenic claudication and, 36
Seronegative arthropathies, 65–66
Shoes, 117, 121
    metatarsal bars inserted into, 122–123
Shoulders, 40–55
    adhesive capsulitis, 49–50
    aging and, 41
    anatomy and function of, 40–41
    arthritis in, 50
    avascular necrosis, 52
    bicipital tendinitis, 48–49
    calcific tendinitis, 47–48
    causes of pain, *42*
    clinical assessment, 42–43
    diagram of, *41*
    extrinsic disorders of, 52–54
    fibrositis, 51–52

intrinsic disorders, 45–52
Milwaukee shoulder syndrome, 50–51
myopathies involving, 53
neck references to, 21
neoplasms, 52
neurogenic pain, 53–54
neurovascular pain, 54
pain management regimen, *46*
polymyalgia rheumatica, 53
radiographic investigations, 43–44
range of motion of, *44*
reflex dystrophy, 54
rotator cuff lesions, 45–46
rotator cuff ruptures, 48
shoulder-hand syndrome, 69
systemic or generalized arthritis involving, 52–53
viscerosomatic pain, 53
Smoking, osteoporosis and, 92
Social work, in dysmobility rehabilitation, 136
Sodium fluoride, osteoporosis managed with, 93–94
Soft cervical collars, 22
Soft-tissue rheumatism, 12
Spinal stenosis, 35–39
    decompressive lumbar laminectomy to treat, 38
    diagnosis of, 35–36
    neurogenic claudication associated with, 36–37
Splayfoot, 121–123
Splints, in carpal tunnel syndrome management, 61
Sprains, ankle, 116–117
Staphylococci, sepsis due to, 111–112
Stenosing tenosynovitis, 61–62
    in wrists, 62–63
Stenosis, *see* Spinal stenosis
Sternoclavicular joint, of shoulder, 40
Stroke, 11, 131–132
Subcutaneous fatpad, loss of, 116
Subtaler joints, 117
    motion range of, 113–114
Synovectomy, 114
Synovial fluid
    in hip, 87
    immune complexes deposited as, 2
    in Milwaukee shoulder syndrome, 51
    uric acid and calcium pyrophosphate distinguished in, 7
Systemic lupus erythematosus, 65–66
    osteonecrosis and, 89

T
Tailor's bunion, 121
Temporal arteritis, 13
Tenderness, pain distinguished from, 99
Tendinitis, 14, 73
    Achilles, 115